# Now I Lay Me Down To Sleep

SECOND EDITION

*A Ministry Resource For Hospice Patients And Their Caregivers…*

Compiled by
Bonnie Evans

*Legacies,*
*preserving the memories of ordinary people*
Ione, California

Cover design by Amos of Fiverr.



For more information about copyright permission:
Bonnie Evans
bonniere@gmail.com


ISBN: 978-0-9915634-7-0

**Dedicated**
**to those seeking peace and rest**
**in their final days …**
**and to the loved ones**
**who watch over and wait with them.**

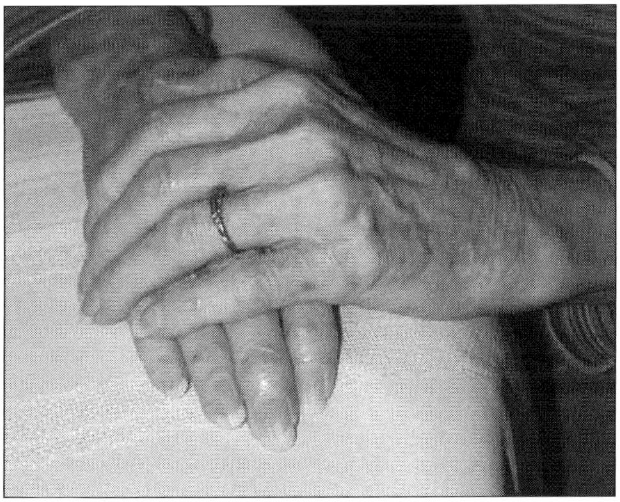

***Now I lay me down to sleep,***
***I pray the Lord my soul to keep.***
***If I should die before I wake,***
***I pray the Lord my soul to take.***
***Amen.***

# Contents

# Preface

As with many philanthropic endeavors, *Now I Lay Me Down To Sleep* wasn't born overnight ....

**For thirteen years,** I volunteered for a hospice program as a respite caregiver (sitting with terminally ill patients to give their full-time caregivers a chance to relax or run errands). God gave me the grace to show up, be present, listen, talk, or just sit with them in silence.

Throughout those years, I watched patients and their caregivers struggle through the well-documented 'agitation phase of dying'—the stage where the patient is restless, agitated, plucking covers, trying to get out of bed, and sometimes hallucinating. There is medication to alleviate those symptoms, but one of my patients used a much less invasive way to address it in an even more effective way.

When I was with Nan during a period of apprehension, she'd ask me to read from her Bible or sing hymns. She usually requested specific scriptures—and, I've never been much of a singer, but did my best to sing every scripture chorus and hymn I knew when asked. Every time we began her ritual, I saw immediate relief spread through her countenance and physical being.

As a first-person witness to her need and resolution, I became a participant in the solution. It worked instantly for her. I wondered how I could help others follow her path to peace.

I decided to handwrite and carry Bible verses to every household visit in case another patient made the same request. It didn't take long to realize I needed to type and bind my collection so it was easier to find things and keep the pages in order. Every time I used them, I witnessed the Word of God do its work.

Over time, I also heard stories from caregivers who had unsuccessfully searched for a meaningful scripture during a long, hard night. The idea of leaving Bible Verse Booklets with families began to form.

Since Nan often requested a Psalm, I started searching the Bible's songbook for words that might comfort hospice patients and caregivers. Then, I turned to other Biblical books offering encouragement. As I collected them, I sorted them into the five themes hospice patients often need to express or hear (I Am Loved, Thank You, I Need You, Forgive Me, I Forgive You).

When I felt confident of the Bible verses I'd accumulated, I looked for well-known hymns that echoed those messages of peace and comfort and inserted them throughout the manuscript. Section One of this book is filled with those verses and hymns. Although this is not the first or only book with scriptures arranged by topic, it was prepared in large, bold print for easy reading.

**As the project came to a close, I had another idea** .... As a San Jose State graduate student, I conducted life reviews with terminally ill patients and/or their caregivers. After each interview, I typed and modified all of the pages by editing, organizing, and inserting personal photographs. Each family received a bound copy of their interview for themselves and their descendants.

As I put the final touches on *Now I Lay Me Down To Sleep*, it occurred to me that many of those stories had the potential to encourage others involved in hospice care. I asked participants if they'd consent to have portions of their interviews anonymously included in this book. Everyone agreed. [The questions I used for those interviews are included on pages 125-128.]

**The prototype of *Now I Lay Me Down To Sleep*** was published in March of 2007. They were printed and spiral-bound in my home office.

In 2017, I discovered a website that would professionally print and bind the books for a reasonable fee. I decided to copyright it and make it available on Amazon and in bookstores. To keep the cost of the book reasonable, I only used black-and-white photography.

**The SECOND EDITION of *Now I Lay Me Down To Sleep*** was published in June 2025. The 2017 edition was edited and amended in the following ways:

- The work in Section One was originally based on the Revised Standard Version of the Bible; the SECOND edition includes scriptures from five different versions. The version is cited with each scripture.

- The testimonies in Section Two were originally from my San Jose State Thesis project and had to remain anonymous. The SECOND edition includes interviews and short stories from friends who have walked in the role of caregiver to a hospice patient after I graduated. They signed consent forms and asked to be identified.

It has been a blessing to compile and publish both editions. I pray the blessing will extend to you as well. When you no longer need your copy of *Now I Lay Me Down To Sleep*, I hope you'll pass it on or leave it where it has the potential to be used.

Bonnie Evans
*Legacies*, Preserving Memories of Ordinary People
Ione, California

# Section One—
## *Bible Verses*

In our final days on this side of heaven, it's normal to experience episodes of mild to severe agitation during the dying process. The accepted medical response to this type of end-stage restlessness is medication.

I know drugs for end-of-life symptoms are effective. I have discovered another (less invasive) means to resolve physical and emotional distress: Reading the Word of God out loud. It's inexpensive, powerful, and simple.

If you're going to read to someone from the following pages (or scriptures of your choosing), read slowly and softly. Pause often to let the power of the words do their work. It doesn't matter if the listener is awake or in a state of restless sleep—I promise you—God's Words will bear the fruit of peace in your patient.

This strategy can also be used with dementia or Alzheimer's patients who are restless and agitated. The Word of God has the power to soothe souls. It can be addictive, but it is never unnecessary.

The Bible verses are divided into the five general themes terminal patients most often feel the need to hear or say:

- I Am Loved
- Thank You
- I Need You
- Forgive Me
- I Forgive You

If you don't sense your loved one has a specific need, read from any of the first three categories.

# Scriptures

**Forever, O LORD, thy word is firmly fixed in the heavens.** Psalm 119:89 [RSV]

**Thy word is a lamp to my feet and a light to my path.** Psalm 119:105 [RSV]

**Every word of God proves true; he is a shield to those who take refuge in him.** Proverbs 30:5 [RSV]

**All scripture is inspired by God and profitable for teaching, for reproof, for correction, and for training in righteousness, that the man of God may be complete, equipped for every good work.** 2 Timothy 3:16-17 [RSV]

**For the word of God is living and active, sharper than any two-edged sword, piercing to the division of soul and spirit, of joints and marrow, and discerning the thoughts and intentions of the heart.** Hebrews 4:12 [RSV]

In the first edition of this book, all Bible verses were typed from the Revised Standard Version (RSV) of the Bible. The reason was personal … I was raised in a Christian home, in the Lutheran Church, and required to memorize hundreds of Bible verses. All of them were in the King James voice. When I bought my first study Bible at the age of 25, I looked for a version that would resonate with the vocabulary I'd memorized as a child. To this day, when I'm looking to use the Word for teaching or as a weapon of warfare, I turn to the Bible which sounds most like the words God stored in my heart years ago.

In the SECOND EDITION, I used five different versions of the verses: Revised Standard Version (RSV), New King James Version (NKJV), King James Version (KJV), New International Version (NIV), and The Message Bible (MSG).

NOTE: For *Gratis Use*, the words and punctuation must be exactly as they appear in the translation. Which means the punctuation, spelling, capital letters, etc., will vary from scripture to scripture.

# I Am Loved

***"We love because He first loved us."*** 1 John 4:19 [RSV]

## ***Psalm 23*** [KJV]

**1 The LORD is my shepherd; I shall not want.**

**2 He maketh me to lie down in green pastures: he leadeth me beside the still waters.**

**3 He restoreth my soul: he leadeth me in the paths of righteousness for his name's sake.**

**4 Yea, though I walk through the valley of the shadow of death, I will fear no evil: for thou art with me; thy rod and thy staff they comfort me.**

**5 Thou preparest a table before me in the presence of mine enemies: thou anointest my head with oil; my cup runneth over.**

**6 Surely goodness and mercy shall follow me all the days of my life: and I will dwell in the house of the LORD for ever.**

"For God so loved the world that He gave His only begotten Son, that whoever believes in Him should not perish but have everlasting life." John 3:16 [NKJV]

## ***Psalm 8*** [NKJV]

**1 O Lord, our Lord, How excellent is Your name in all the earth,**
**Who have set Your glory above the heavens!**

**2 Out of the mouth of babes and nursing infants You have ordained strength, Because of Your enemies, That You may silence the enemy and the avenger.**

**3 When I consider Your heavens, the work of Your fingers, The**
**moon and the stars, which You have ordained, 4 What is man**
**that You are mindful of him, And the son of man that You**
**visit him?**

**5 For You have made him a little lower than the angels, And You**
**have crowned him with glory and honor. 6 You have made**
**him to have dominion over the works of Your hands; You**
**have put all things under his feet, 7 All sheep and oxen—**
**Even the beasts of the field, 8 The birds of the air, And the**
**fish of the sea That pass through the paths of the seas.**

**9 O Lord, our Lord, How excellent is Your name in all the earth!**

## ***John 10*** [*portions*, NKJV]

**11 I am the good shepherd. The good shepherd gives His life for the sheep.**

. . . . . .

**14 I am the good shepherd; and I know My sheep, and am known by**
**My own. 15 As the Father knows Me, even so I know the Father; and**
**I lay down My life for the sheep.**

. . . . .

**17 Therefore My Father loves Me, because I lay down My life that I**
**may take it again. 18 No one takes it from Me, but I lay it down of**
**Myself. I have power to lay it down, and I have power to take it**
**again. This command I have received from My Father.**

## ***Psalm 18*** [*portions*, KJV]

**1 I will love thee, O LORD, my strength. 2 The LORD is my rock,
and my fortress, and my deliverer; my God, my strength, in whom I
will trust 3 my God, my strength, in whom I will trust; my buckler,
and the horn of my salvation, and my high tower.**

**3 I will call upon the LORD, who is worthy to be praised: so shall I
be saved from mine enemies.**

**4 The sorrows of death compassed me, and the floods of ungodly men
made me afraid. 5 The sorrows of hell compassed me about:
the snares of death prevented me. 6 In my distress I called upon the
LORD, and cried unto my God: he heard my voice out of his temple,
and my cry came before him, even into his ears.**

. . . . .

**28 For thou wilt light my candle: the LORD my God will enlighten my
darkness. 29 For by thee I have run through a troop; and by my God
have I leaped over a wall.**

**30 As for God, his way is perfect: the word of the LORD is tried: he is
a buckler to all those that trust in him. 31 For who is God save the
LORD? or who is a rock save our God?**

**32 It is God that girdeth me with strength, and maketh my way
perfect. 33 He maketh my feet like hinds' feet, and setteth me upon
my high places. 34 He teacheth my hands to war, so that a bow of
steel is broken by mine arms.**

**35 Thou hast also given me the shield of thy salvation: and thy right
hand hath holden me up, and thy gentleness hath made me great.
36 Thou hast enlarged my steps under me, that my feet did not slip.**

. . . . .

**46 The LORD liveth; and blessed be my rock; and let the God of my
salvation be exalted. 47 It is God that avengeth me, and subdueth the
people under me. 48 He delivereth me from mine enemies: yea, thou
liftest me up above those that rise up against me: thou hast delivered
me from the violent man. 49 Therefore will I give thanks unto thee,
O LORD, among the heathen, and sing praises unto thy name.**

## ***Psalm 20*** [NIV]

**1 May the LORD answer you when you are in distress; may**
**the name of the God of Jacob protect you. 2 May he**
**send you help from the sanctuary and grant you support**
**from Zion. 3 May he remember all your sacrifices and**
**accept your burnt offerings. 4 May he give you the**
**desire of your heart and make all your plans succeed.**

**5 May we shout for joy over your victory and lift up our**
**banners in the name of our God. May the LORD grant**
**all your requests.**

**6 Now this I know: The LORD gives victory to his anointed.**
**He answers him from his heavenly sanctuary with the**
**victorious power of his right hand. 7 Some trust in**
**chariots and some in horses, but we trust in the name of**
**the LORD our God. 8 They are brought to their knees**
**and fall, but we rise up and stand firm.**

**9 LORD, give victory to the king! Answer us when we call!**

## ***Psalm 32:6-7*** [RSV]

**6 Therefore let every one who is godly**
**offer prayer to thee;**
**at a time of distress,**
**in the rush of great waters,**
**they shall not reach him.**

**7 Thou art a hiding place for me,**
**thou preservest me from trouble;**
**thou dost encompass me with deliverance.**

"God is love…"

1 John 4:16
KJV

## ***Psalm 46:10*** [RSV]

**"Be still, and know that I am God."**

## ***Psalm 24*** [*portions*, NIV]

**1 The earth is the LORD's, and everything in it, the
world, and all who live in it; 2 for he founded it on the
seas and established it on the waters.**

. . . . .

**7 Lift up your heads, you gates; be lifted up, you
ancient doors, that the King of glory may come in.**

**8 Who is this King of glory? The LORD strong and
mighty, the LORD mighty in battle.**

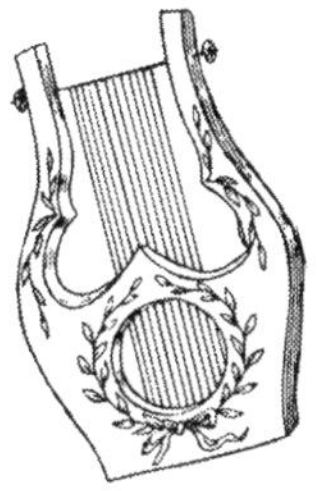

**9 Lift up your heads, you gates; lift them up, you
ancient doors, that the King of glory may come in.**

**10 Who is he, this King of glory? The LORD
Almighty— he is the King of glory.**

## ***Psalm 33*** [*portions*, NIV]

**1 Sing joyfully to the LORD, you righteous; it is fitting for the upright
to praise him. 2 Praise the LORD with the harp; make music to him
on the ten-stringed lyre. 3 Sing to him a new song; play skillfully, and
shout for joy.**

**4 For the word of the LORD is right and true; he is faithful in all he
does. 5 The LORD loves righteousness and justice; the earth is full of
his unfailing love.**

. . . . .

**18 But the eyes of the LORD are on those who fear him, on those
whose hope is in his unfailing love, 19 to deliver them from death and
keep them alive in famine.**

**20 We wait in hope for the LORD; he is our help and our shield.
21 In him our hearts rejoice, for we trust in his holy name. 22 May
your unfailing love be with us, LORD, even as we put our hope in
you.**

## *Psalm 27* [KJV]

**1 The LORD is my light and my salvation; whom shall I fear? The LORD is the strength of my life; of whom shall I be afraid?**

**2 When the wicked, even mine enemies and my foes, came upon me
to eat up my flesh, they stumbled and fell. 3 Though an host
should encamp against me, my heart shall not fear: though
war should rise against me, in this will I be confident.**

**4 One thing have I desired of the LORD, that will I seek after; that I may dwell in the house of the LORD all the days of my life, to behold the beauty of the LORD, and to enquire in his temple.**

**5 For in the time of trouble he shall hide me in his pavilion: in the secret of his tabernacle shall he hide me; he shall set me up upon a rock.**

**6 And now shall mine head be lifted up above mine enemies round about me: therefore will I offer in his tabernacle sacrifices of joy; I will sing, yea, I will sing praises unto the LORD.**

**7 Hear, O LORD, when I cry with my voice: have mercy also upon
me, and answer me. 8 When thou saidst, Seek ye my face;
my heart said unto thee, Thy face, LORD, will I seek.**

**9 Hide not thy face far from me; put not thy servant away in anger:
thou hast been my help; leave me not, neither forsake me, O
God of my salvation. 10 When my father and my mother
forsake me, then the LORD will take me up.**

**11 Teach me thy way, O LORD, and lead me in a plain path,
because of mine enemies. 12 Deliver me not over unto the will
of mine enemies: for false witnesses are risen up against me,
and such as breathe out cruelty. 13 I had fainted, unless I had
believed to see the goodness of the LORD in the land of the
living.**

**14 Wait on the LORD: be of good courage, and he shall strengthen thine heart: wait, I say, on the LORD.**

## *1 Corinthians 13:8-13* [RSV]

**8 Love never ends; as for prophecies, they will pass
away; as for tongues, they will cease; as for knowledge,
it will pass away.**

**9 For our knowledge is imperfect and our prophecy is
imperfect; 10 but when the perfect comes, the imperfect
will pass away.**

**11 When I was a child, I spoke like a child, I thought
like a child, I reasoned like a child; when I became a
man, I gave up childish ways.**

**12 For now we see in a mirror dimly, but then face to
face. Now I know in part; then I shall understand
fully, even as I have been fully understood.**

**13 So faith, hope, love abide, these three; but the
greatest of these is love.**

## *Psalm 29:1-4, 10-11* [RSV]

**1 Ascribe to the LORD, O heavenly beings, ascribe to the
LORD glory and strength. 2 Ascribe to the LORD the
glory of his name; worship the LORD in holy array.**

**3 The voice of the LORD is upon the waters; the God of glory
thunders, the LORD, upon many waters. 4 The voice of the
LORD is powerful, the voice of the LORD is full of majesty.**

. . . . .

**10 The LORD sits enthroned over the flood;
the LORD sits enthroned as king for ever.**

**11 May the LORD give strength to his people!**

**May the LORD bless his people with peace!**

## *Psalm 52:8-9* [NKJV]

**8 But I am like a green olive tree in the house of God; I trust in the mercy of God forever and ever.**

**9 I will praise You forever, Because You have done it; And in the presence of Your saints I will wait on Your name, for it is good.**

## *Psalm 49:5-8* [NKJV]

**5 Why should I fear in the days of evil,**
**When the iniquity at my heels surrounds me?**

**6 Those who trust in their wealth and boast in the multitude of their**
**riches, 7 None of them can by any means redeem his brother, Nor**
**give to God a ransom for him—8 For the redemption of their**
**souls is costly, And it shall cease forever.**

## *Psalm 72:18-19* [KJV]

**18 Blessed be the LORD God, the God of Israel, who only doeth wondrous things.**

**19 And blessed be his glorious name for ever: and let the whole earth be filled with his glory; Amen, and Amen.**

## *Psalm 65:1-4* [MSG]

**1 Silence is praise to you, Zion-dwelling God, and also obedience.**

**2 You hear the prayer in it all. We all arrive at your doorstep sooner**
**or later, loaded with guilt, 3 Our sins too much for us—but you get**
**rid of them once and for all.**

**4 Blessed are the chosen! Blessed the guest at home in your place! We expect our fill of good things in your house, your heavenly manse.**

## ***Psalm 34*** [*portions*, NKJV]

**1 I will bless the Lord at all times; His praise shall continually be in**
**my mouth. 2 My soul shall make its boast in the Lord; The humble**
**shall hear of it and be glad.**

**3 Oh, magnify the Lord with me, And let us exalt His name together.**
**4 I sought the Lord, and He heard me, And delivered me from all my**
**fears. 5 They looked to Him and were radiant, And their faces were**
**not ashamed. 6 This poor man cried out, And the Lord heard him,**
**And saved him out of all his troubles.**

**7 The angel of the Lord encamps all around those who fear Him, And**
**delivers them. 8 Oh, taste and see that the Lord is good; Blessed is**
**the man who trusts in Him! 9 Oh, fear the Lord, you His saints!**
**There is no want to those who fear Him.**

. . . . .

**15 The eyes of the Lord are on the righteous, And His ears are open to**
**their cry. 16 The face of the Lord is against those who do evil,**
**To cut off the remembrance of them from the earth.**
**17 The righteous cry out, and the Lord hears, And delivers them out**
**of all their troubles. 18 The Lord is near to those who have a broken**
**heart, And saves such as have a contrite spirit. 19 Many are the**
**afflictions of the righteous, But the Lord delivers him out of them all.**

. . . . .

**22 The Lord redeems the soul of His servants,**
**And none of those who trust in Him shall be condemned.**

## ***Psalm 59:16-17*** [NKJV]

**16 But I will sing of Your power; Yes, I will sing aloud of Your mercy in the morning; For You have been my defense and refuge in the day of my trouble.**

**17 To You, O my Strength, I will sing praises; For God is my defense, My God of mercy.**

***Psalm 37*** [*portions*, NKJV]

**4 Delight yourself also in the Lord, And He shall give you the desires of your heart.**

**5 Commit your way to the Lord, Trust also in Him, And He shall**
**bring it to pass. 6 He shall bring forth your righteousness as**
**the light, And your justice as the noonday.**

**7 Rest in the Lord, and wait patiently for Him; Do not fret because of him who prospers in his way, Because of the man who brings wicked schemes to pass.**

**8 Cease from anger, and forsake wrath; Do not fret— it only causes harm.**

. . . . .

**23 The steps of a good man are ordered by the Lord, And He delights**
**in his way. 24 Though he fall, he shall not be utterly cast down;**
**For the Lord upholds him with His hand.**

**25 I have been young, and now am old; Yet I have not seen the righteous forsaken, Nor his descendants begging bread.**

**26 He is ever merciful, and lends; And his descendants are blessed.**

. . . . .

**28 For the Lord loves justice, And does not forsake His saints; They**
**are preserved forever, But the descendants of the wicked shall be cut**
**off. 29 The righteous shall inherit the land, And dwell in it forever.**

**30 The mouth of the righteous speaks wisdom, And his tongue talks**
**of justice. 31 The law of his God is in his heart; None of his steps**
**shall slide.**

"For I am persuaded, that neither death, nor life, nor angels, nor principalities, nor powers, nor things present, nor things to come, Nor height, nor depth, nor any other creature, shall be able to separate us from the love of God, which is in Christ Jesus our Lord." Romans 8:38, 39 [KJV]

## ***Psalm 42*** [NIV]

1 **As the deer pants for streams of water, so my soul pants for you,**
**my God.** 2 **My soul thirsts for God, for the living God.**
**When can I go and meet with God?**

3 **My tears have been my food day and night, while people say to me all day long, "Where is your God?"**

4 **These things I remember as I pour out my soul: how I used to go to the house of God under the protection of the Mighty One with shouts of joy and praise among the festive throng.**

5 **Why, my soul, are you downcast? Why so disturbed within me? Put your hope in God, for I will yet praise him, my Savior and my God.**

6 **My soul is downcast within me; therefore I will remember you from the land of the Jordan, the heights of Hermon—from Mount Mizar.**

7 **Deep calls to deep in the roar of your waterfalls; all your waves and breakers have swept over me.**

8 **By day the LORD directs his love, at night his song is with me— a prayer to the God of my life.**

9 **I say to God my Rock, "Why have you forgotten me? Why must I go about mourning, oppressed by the enemy?"**

10 **My bones suffer mortal agony as my foes taunt me, saying to me all day long, "Where is your God?"**

11 **Why, my soul, are you downcast? Why so disturbed within me? Put your hope in God, for I will yet praise him, my Savior and my God.**

"But we have this treasure in earthen vessels, to show that the transcendent power belongs to God and not to us.
We are afflicted in every way, but not crushed; perplexed, but not driven to despair; persecuted, but not forsaken; struck down, but not destroyed..." 2 Corinthians 4:7-9 [RSV]

## ***Psalm 46*** [NKJV]

1 God is our refuge and strength, A very present help in trouble.
2 Therefore we will not fear, Even though the earth be
removed, And though the mountains be carried into the
midst of the sea; 3 Though its waters roar and be troubled,
Though the mountains shake with its swelling. Selah

4 There is a river whose streams shall make glad the city of God,
The holy place of the tabernacle of the Most High. 5 God is in
the midst of her, she shall not be moved; God shall help her,
just at the break of dawn. 6 The nations raged, the kingdoms
were moved; He uttered His voice, the earth melted. 7 The
Lord of hosts is with us; The God of Jacob is our refuge. Selah

8 Come, behold the works of the Lord, Who has made desolations
in the earth. 9 He makes wars cease to the end of the earth;
He breaks the bow and cuts the spear in two; He burns the
chariot in the fire.

10 Be still, and know that I am God; I will be exalted among the
nations, I will be exalted in the earth!

11 The Lord of hosts is with us; The God of Jacob is our refuge. Selah

## ***Psalm 81:1-2, 5-7*** [NIV]

1 Sing for joy to God our strength;
shout aloud to the God of Jacob!
2 Begin the music, strike the timbrel,
play the melodious harp and lyre.

. . . . .

5 When God went out against Egypt, he established it as a statute for
Joseph. I heard an unknown voice say: 6 "I removed the burden
from their shoulders; their hands were set free from the basket.
7 In your distress you called and I rescued you, I answered you
out of a thundercloud; I tested you at the waters of Meribah."

"Therefore we do not lose heart. Though outwardly we are wasting away, yet inwardly we are being renewed day by day.

For our light and momentary troubles are achieving for us an eternal glory that far outweighs them all.

So we fix our eyes not on what is seen, but on what is unseen, since what is seen is temporary, but what is unseen is eternal."

2 Corinthians 4:16-18 [NIV]

## ***Psalm 84*** [NIV]

**1 How lovely is your dwelling place, LORD Almighty! 2 My soul**
**yearns, even faints, for the courts of the LORD; my heart**
**and my flesh cry out for the living God.**

**3 Even the sparrow has found a home, and the swallow a nest for**
**herself, where she may have her young—a place near your**
**altar, LORD Almighty, my King and my God.**

**4 Blessed are those who dwell in your house; they are ever praising**
**you. 5 Blessed are those whose strength is in you, whose hearts**
**are set on pilgrimage. 6 As they pass through the Valley of**
**Baka, they make it a place of springs; the autumn rains also**
**cover it with pools. 7 They go from strength to strength, till**
**each appears before God in Zion.**

**8 Hear my prayer, LORD God Almighty; listen to me, God of Jacob.**

**9 Look on our shield, O God; look with favor on your anointed one.**

**10 Better is one day in your courts than a thousand elsewhere;**
**I would rather be a doorkeeper in the house of my God**
**than dwell in the tents of the wicked.**

**11 For the LORD God is a sun and shield; the LORD bestows**
**favor and honor; no good thing does he withhold from**
**those whose walk is blameless.**

**12 LORD Almighty, blessed is the one who trusts in you.**

## ***Psalm 89*** [*portions*, RSV]

**1 I will sing of thy steadfast love, O LORD, for ever; with my mouth**
**I will proclaim thy faithfulness to all generations. 2 For thy**
**steadfast love was established for ever, thy faithfulness is**
**firm as the heavens.**

. . . . .

**5 Let the heavens praise thy wonders, O LORD, thy faithfulness in**
**the assembly of the holy ones! 6 For who in the skies can be**
**compared to the LORD? Who among the heavenly beings is**
**like the LORD, 7 a God feared in the council of the holy ones,**
**great and terrible above all that are round about him? 8 O**
**LORD God of hosts, who is mighty as thou art, O LORD,**
**with thy faithfulness round about thee?**

. . . . .

**13 Thou hast a mighty arm; strong is thy hand, high thy right hand.**
**14 Righteousness and justice are the foundation of thy throne;**
**steadfast love and faithfulness go before thee.**

**15 Blessed are the people who know the festal shout, who walk, O**
**LORD, in the light of thy countenance, 16 who exult in thy**
**name all the day, and extol thy righteousness.**

**17 For thou art the glory of their strength; by thy favor our horn is**
**exalted. 18 For our shield belongs to the LORD, our king**
**to the Holy One of Israel.**

## ***Psalm 96:1-4a*** [MSG]

**1 Sing God a brand-new song! Earth and everyone in it, sing!**

**2 Sing to God—worship God! Shout the news of his victory from sea**
**to sea, 3 Take the news of his glory to the lost, News of his wonders to**
**one and all! 4 For God is great, and worth a thousand Hallelujahs ....**

## ***Psalm 93*** [MSG]

**1 God is King, robed and ruling, God is robed and surging with**
**strength. And yes, the world is firm, immovable, 2 Your throne**
**ever firm—you're Eternal!**

**3 Sea storms are up, God, Sea storms wild and roaring, Sea storms**
**with thunderous breakers. 4 Stronger than wild sea storms, Mightier**
**than sea-storm breakers, Mighty God rules from High Heaven.**

**5 What you say goes—it always has. "Beauty" and "Holy" mark**
**your palace rule, God, to the very end of time.**

## ***Psalm 100*** [RSV]

**1 Make a joyful noise to the LORD, all the lands! 2 Serve the**
**LORD with gladness! Come into his presence with singing!**

**3 Know that the LORD is God! It is he that made us, and we**
**are his; we are his people, and the sheep of his pasture.**

**4 Enter his gates with thanksgiving, and his courts with praise!**
**Give thanks to him, bless his name!**

**5 For the LORD is good; his steadfast love endures for ever,**
**and his faithfulness to all generations.**

## ***Psalm 117*** [RSV]

**1 Praise the LORD, all nations! Extol him, all peoples! 2 For great is**
**his steadfast love toward us; and the faithfulness of the LORD**
**endures for ever. Praise the LORD!**

"... thank God no matter what happens. This is the way God wants you who belong to Christ Jesus to live." 1 Thessalonians 5:18 [MSG]

## ***Psalm 90*** [*portions*, NKJV]

**1 A Prayer of Moses the man of God. Lord, You have been our
dwelling place in all generations. 2 Before the mountains were
brought forth, Or ever You had formed the earth and the
world, Even from everlasting to everlasting, You are God.**

. . . . .

**12 So teach us to number our days, That we may gain a heart of
wisdom.**

**13 Return, O Lord! How long? And have compassion on Your
servants. 14 Oh, satisfy us early with Your mercy, That we may
rejoice and be glad all our days! 15 Make us glad according to
the days in which You have afflicted us, The years in which we
have seen evil.**

**16 Let Your work appear to Your servants, And Your glory to their
children. 17 And let the beauty of the Lord our God be upon us,
And establish the work of our hands for us; Yes, establish the
work of our hands.**

## ***Psalm 95:1-7*** [KJV]

**1 O come, let us sing unto the LORD: let us make a joyful noise to the
rock of our salvation. 2 Let us come before his presence with
thanksgiving, and make a joyful noise unto him with psalms.**

**3 For the LORD is a great God, and a great King above all
gods. 4 In his hand are the deep places of the earth: the
strength of the hills is his also. 5 The sea is his, and he
made it: and his hands formed the dry land.**

**6 O come, let us worship and bow down: let us kneel before the
LORD our maker. 7 For he is our God; and we are the people of his
pasture, and the sheep of his hand. Today if ye will hear his voice, for
his hands formed the dry land.**

## ***Psalm 98:1-5*** [KJV]

**1 O sing unto the LORD a new song; for he hath done marvellous things: his right hand, and his holy arm, hath gotten him the victory.**

**2 The LORD hath made known his salvation: his righteousness hath he openly shewed in the sight of the heathen.**

**3 He hath remembered his mercy and his truth toward the house of Israel: all the ends of the earth have seen the salvation of our God.**

**4 Make a joyful noise unto the LORD, all the earth: make a loud noise, and rejoice, and sing praise.**

**5 Sing unto the LORD with the harp; with the harp, and the voice of a psalm.**

> *"See those people polishing their chariots, and those others grooming their horses? But we're making garlands for God our God. The chariots will rust, those horses pull up lame - and we'll be on our feet, standing tall. Make the king a winner, God; the day we call, give us your answer."* Psalm 20:7-8 [MSG]

## ***Psalm 115:1-9*** [KJV]

**1 Not unto us, O LORD, not unto us, but unto thy name give glory, for thy mercy, and for thy truth's sake.**

**2 Wherefore should the heathen say, Where is now their God?**

**3 But our God is in the heavens: he hath done whatsoever he hath pleased.**

**4 Their idols are silver and gold, the work of**
**men's hands. 5 They have mouths, but they**
**speak not: eyes have they, but they see not:**
**6 They have ears, but they hear not: noses**
**have they, but they smell not: 7 They have**
**hands, but they handle not: feet have they,**
**but they walk not: neither speak they**
**through their throat.**

**8 They that make them are like unto them; so is every one that trusteth in them.**

**9 O Israel, trust thou in the LORD: he is their help and their shield.**

## *Psalm 134* [RSV]

1 **Come, bless the LORD, all you servants of the LORD, who stand by night in the house of the LORD!**

2 **Lift up your hands to the holy place, and bless the LORD!**

3 **May the LORD bless you from Zion, he who made heaven and earth!**

TRUST

## *Psalm 125:1-2* [RSV]

1 **Those who trust in the LORD are like Mount Zion, which cannot be moved, but abides for ever.**

2 **As the mountains are round about Jerusalem, so the LORD is round about his people, from this time forth and for evermore.**

## *Psalm 140:12-13* [RSV]

12 **I know that the LORD maintains the cause of the afflicted,**
**and executes justice for the needy.**

13 **Surely the righteous shall give thanks to thy name;**
**the upright shall dwell in thy presence.**

## *Psalm 135* [*portions*, KJV]

5 **For I know that the LORD is great, and that our Lord is above all**
**gods. 6 Whatsoever the LORD pleased, that did he in heaven, and in**
**earth, in the seas, and all deep places. 7 He causeth the vapours to**
**ascend from the ends of the earth; he maketh lightnings for the rain;**
**he bringeth the wind out of his treasuries.**

. . . . .

13 **Thy name, O LORD, endureth for ever; and thy memorial, O LORD, throughout all generations.**

## ***Psalm 103*** *[portions,* NIV]

**1 Praise the LORD, my soul; all my inmost being, praise his holy
name. 2 Praise the LORD, my soul, and forget not all his
benefits—3 who forgives all your sins and heals all your
diseases, 4 who redeems your life from the pit and crowns you
with love and compassion, 5 who satisfies your desires with
good things so that your youth is renewed like the eagle's.**

**6 The LORD works righteousness and justice for all the oppressed.**

**7 He made known his ways to Moses, his deeds to the people of Israel:
8 The LORD is compassionate and gracious, slow to anger,
abounding in love.**

**9 He will not always accuse, nor will he harbor his anger forever;
10 he does not treat us as our sins deserve or repay us according
to our iniquities.**

**11 For as high as the heavens are above the earth, so great is his love
for those who fear him; 12 as far as the east is from the west,
so far has he removed our transgressions from us.**

**13 As a father has compassion on his children, so the LORD has
compassion on those who fear him; 14 for he knows how we
are formed, he remembers that we are dust.**

**15 The life of mortals is like grass, they flourish like a flower of the
field; 16 the wind blows over it and it is gone, and its place
remembers it no more.**

**17 But from everlasting to everlasting the LORD's love is with those
who fear him, and his righteousness with their children's
children—18 with those who keep his covenant and remember
to obey his precepts.**

. . . . .

**20 Praise the LORD, you his angels, you mighty ones who do his
bidding, who obey his word. 21 Praise the LORD, all his
heavenly hosts, you his servants who do his will.**

**22 Praise the LORD, all his works everywhere in his dominion.
Praise the LORD, my soul.**

## *Psalm 104* [*portions*, NIV]

**1 Praise the LORD, my soul. LORD my God, you are very**
**great; you are clothed with splendor and majesty.**

**2 The LORD wraps himself in light as with a garment; he**
**stretches out the heavens like a tent 3 and lays the beams**
**of his upper chambers on their waters. He makes the**
**clouds his chariot and rides on the wings of the wind.**

**4 He makes winds his messengers, flames of fire his servants.**
**5 He set the earth on its foundations; it can never be**
**moved.**

. . . . .

**24 How many are your works, LORD! In wisdom you made**
**them all; the earth is full of your creatures.**

**25 There is the sea, vast and spacious, teeming with creatures**
**beyond number—living things both large and small.**
**26 There the ships go to and fro, and Leviathan, which**
**you formed to frolic there.**

**27 All creatures look to you to give them their food at the**
**proper time. 28 When you give it to them, they gather**
**it up; when you open your hand, they are satisfied with**
**good things. 29 When you hide your face, they are**
**terrified; when you take away their breath, they die and**
**return to the dust. 30 When you send your Spirit, they**
**are created, and you renew the face of the ground.**

**31 May the glory of the LORD endure forever; may the LORD**
**rejoice in his works—32 he who looks at the earth, and it**
**trembles, who touches the mountains, and they smoke.**

**33 I will sing to the LORD all my life; I will sing praise to my**
**God as long as I live. 34 May my meditation be pleasing**
**to him, as I rejoice in the LORD.**

## ***Psalm 116*** [NIV]

**1 I love the LORD, for he heard my voice; he heard my cry for
mercy. 2 Because he turned his ear to me, I will call on him
as long as I live.**

**3 The cords of death entangled me, the anguish of the grave came
over me; I was overcome by distress and sorrow.**

**4 Then I called on the name of the LORD: "LORD, save me!"**

**5 The LORD is gracious and righteous; our God is full of compassion.
6 The LORD protects the unwary; when I was brought low, he
saved me.**

**7 Return to your rest, my soul, for the LORD has been good to you.**

**8 For you, LORD, have delivered me from death, my eyes from tears,
my feet from stumbling, 9 that I may walk before the LORD in
the land of the living.**

**10 I trusted in the LORD when I said, "I am greatly afflicted";
11 in my alarm I said, "Everyone is a liar."**

**12 What shall I return to the LORD for all his goodness to me?
13 I will lift up the cup of salvation and call on the name of
the LORD. 14 I will fulfill my vows to the LORD in the
presence of all his people.**

**15 Precious in the sight of the LORD is the death of his faithful
servants.**

**16 Truly I am your servant, LORD; I serve you just as my mother
did; you have freed me from my chains.**

**17 I will sacrifice a thank offering to you and call on the name of the
LORD. 18 I will fulfill my vows to the LORD in the presence
of all his people, 19 in the courts of the house of the LORD—
in your midst, Jerusalem. Praise the LORD.**

"God is striding ahead of you. He's right there with you. He won't let you down; he won't leave you. Don't be intimidated. Don't worry." Deuteronomy 31:8 [MSG]

## ***Psalm 121*** [RSV]

**1 I lift up my eyes to the hills. From whence does my help come?**
**2 My help comes from the LORD, who made heaven and earth.**

**3 He will not let your foot be moved, he who keeps you will not**
**slumber. 4 Behold, he who keeps Israel will neither slumber**
**nor sleep. 5 The LORD is your keeper; the LORD is your**
**shade on your right hand. 6 The sun shall not smite you by day,**
**nor the moon by night.**

**7 The LORD will keep you from all evil; he will keep your life. 8 The**
**LORD will keep your going out and your coming in from this**
**time forth and for evermore.**

## ***Psalm 145*** [*portions*, NKJV]

**1 I will extol You, my God, O King; And I will bless Your name**
**forever and ever. 2 Every day I will bless You, And I will**
**praise Your name forever and ever. 3 Great is the Lord,**
**and greatly to be praised; And His greatness is**
**unsearchable. 4 One generation shall praise Your works**
**to another, And shall declare Your mighty acts.**

. . . . .

**8 The Lord is gracious and full of compassion, Slow to anger**
**and great in mercy. 9 The Lord is good to all, And His**
**tender mercies are over all His works.**

. . . . .

**14 The Lord upholds all who fall, And raises up all who are**
**bowed down. 15 The eyes of all look expectantly to You,**
**And You give them their food in due season. 16 You open**
**Your hand and satisfy the desire of every living thing.**

**17 The Lord is righteous in all His ways, Gracious in all His**
**works. 18 The Lord is near to all who call upon Him,**
**To all who call upon Him in truth. 19 He will fulfill the**
**desire of those who fear Him; He also will hear their cry**
**and save them.**

## ***Psalm 139:1-18*** [RSV]

**1 O LORD, thou hast searched me and known me!**

**2 Thou knowest when I sit down and when I rise up; thou discernest**
**my thoughts from afar. 3 Thou searchest out my path and my**
**lying down, and art acquainted with all my ways.**

**4 Even before a word is on my tongue, lo, O LORD, thou knowest it**
**altogether. 5 Thou dost beset me behind and before, and layest**
**thy hand upon me. 6 Such knowledge is too wonderful for me;**
**it is high, I cannot attain it.**

**7 Whither shall I go from thy Spirit? Or whither shall I flee from thy**
**presence?**

**8 If I ascend to heaven, thou art there! If I make my bed in Sheol,**
**thou art there! 9 If I take the wings of the morning and dwell in**
**the uttermost parts of the sea, 10 even there thy hand shall lead**
**me, and thy right hand shall hold me.**

**11 If I say, "Let only darkness cover me, and the light about me be**
**night," 12 even the darkness is not dark to thee, the night is**
**bright as the day; for darkness is as light with thee.**

**13 For thou didst form my inward parts, thou didst knit me together**
**in my mother's womb.**

**14 I praise thee, for thou art fearful and wonderful. Wonderful are**
**thy works! Thou knowest me right well; 15 my frame was not**
**hidden from thee, when I was being made in secret, intricately**
**wrought in the depths of the earth.**

**16 Thy eyes beheld my unformed substance; in thy book were written,**
**every one of them, the days that were formed for me, when as**
**yet there was none of them.**

**17 How precious to me are thy thoughts, O God! How vast is the sum**
**of them!**

**18 If I would count them, they are more than the sand. When I**
**awake, I am still with thee.**

## ***Psalm 146*** [NKJV]

**1 Praise the Lord! Praise the Lord, O my soul!**

**2 While I live I will praise the Lord; I will sing praises to my**
**God while I have my being.**

**3 Do not put your trust in princes, Nor in a son of man, in**
**whom there is no help. 4 His spirit departs, he returns to**
**his earth; In that very day his plans perish.**

**5 Happy is he who has the God of Jacob for his help, Whose**
**hope is in the Lord his God, 6 Who made heaven and**
**earth, The sea, and all that is in them; Who keeps truth**
**forever, 7 Who executes justice for the oppressed, Who**
**gives food to the hungry. The Lord gives**
**freedom to the prisoners.**

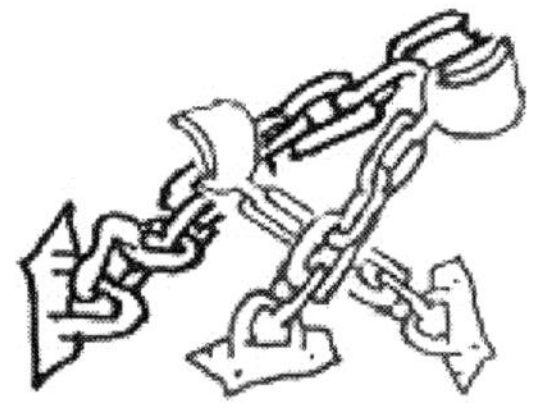

**8 The Lord opens the eyes of the blind; The Lord**
**raises those who are bowed down; The Lord**
**loves the righteous.**

**9 The Lord watches over the strangers; He relieves the**
**fatherless and widow; But the way of the wicked He**
**turns upside down.**

**10 The Lord shall reign forever—Your God, O Zion, to all**
**generations. Praise the Lord!**

## ***Psalm 150:6*** [RSV]

**6 Let everything that breathes praise the LORD! Praise the LORD!**

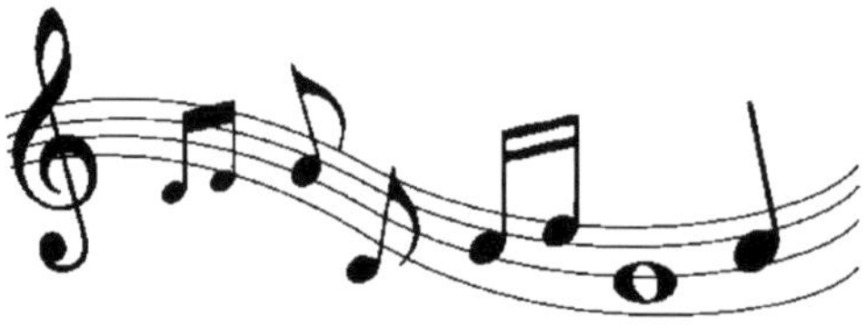

# It Is Well With My Soul

**When Peace like a river attendeth my soul,**
**When sorrows like sea billows roll;**
**Whatever my lot, Thou has taught me to say,**
**It is well, it is well, with my soul.**

**Though Satan should buffet, Though trials should come,**
**Let this blest assurance control,**
**That Christ has regarded my helpless estate,**
**And hath shed His own blood for my soul.**

**My sin, oh, the bliss of this glorious thought!**
**My sin, not in part but the whole,**
**Is nailed to the cross, and I bear it no more,**
**Praise the Lord, Praise the Lord, oh my soul.**

**But, Lord, 'tis for Thee, For Thy coming we wait,**
**The sky, not the grave is our goal.**
**Oh trump of the angel! Oh voice of the Lord!**
**Blessed hope, blessed rest of my soul!**

**And Lord haste the day when my faith shall be sight,**
**The clouds be rolled back as a scroll.**
**The trump shall resound, and the Lord shall descend,**
**Even so, it is well with my soul.**

## CHORUS:

**It is well, with my soul,**
**It is well, with my soul,**
**It is well, it is well, with my soul.**

Written by Horatio Spafford in 1871 … All four of his daughters were killed in a ship accident. When he passed over the spot where they died, the Holy Spirit inspired these words of eternal hope ….

# Jesus Loves Me

**Jesus loves me! This I know,**
**For the Bible tells me so;**
**Little ones to Him belong;**
**They are weak, but He is strong.**

*Refrain:* **Yes, Jesus loves me!**
**Yes, Jesus loves me!**
**Yes, Jesus loves me!**
**The Bible tells me so.**

**Jesus loves me! This I know,**
**As He loved so long ago,**
**Taking children on His knee,**
**Saying, "Let them come to Me."**

**Jesus loves me still today,**
**Walking with me on my way,**
**Wanting as a friend to give**
**Light and love to all who live.**

**Jesus loves me! He who died**
**Heaven's gate to open wide;**
**He will wash away my sin,**
**Let His little child come in.**

**Jesus loves me! He will stay**
**Close beside me all the way;**
**Thou hast bled and died for me,**
**I will henceforth live for Thee.**

"Jesus Loves Me" is a Christian hymn written by Anna Bartlett Warner. The lyrics first appeared as a poem in the context of an 1860 novel called "Say and Seal", written by her older sister Susan Warner (1819-1885). The words were as a poem to a dying child. The tune and refrain were added in 1862 by William Batchelder Bradbury (1816-1868).

# Thank You

***"O give thanks unto the God of heaven: for his mercy endureth for ever."*** Psalm 136:26 [KJV]

"Do not be anxious about anything, but in every situation, by prayer and petition, with thanksgiving, present your requests to God. And the peace of God, which transcends all understanding, will guard your hearts and your minds in Christ Jesus." Philippians 4:6-7 [NIV]

## ***Psalm 4:8*** [NIV]

**8 In peace I will lie down and sleep, for you alone,
LORD, make me dwell in safety.**

## ***Psalm 9*** [*portions*, NIV]

**1 I will give thanks to you, LORD, with all my heart;
I will tell of all your wonderful deeds.**

**2 I will be glad and rejoice in you; I will sing the praises
of your name, O Most High.**

. . . . .

**9 The LORD is a refuge for the oppressed, a stronghold in times of
trouble. 10 Those who know your name trust in you, for you,
LORD, have never forsaken those who seek you. 11 Sing the
praises of the LORD, enthroned in Zion; proclaim among the
nations what he has done.**

## ***Psalm 30:1-5, 11-12*** [NKJV]

**1 I will extol You, O Lord, for You have lifted me up,
And have not let my foes rejoice over me.**

**2 O Lord my God, I cried out to You, And You healed me.
3 O Lord, You brought my soul up from the grave; You have
kept me alive, that I should not go down to the pit.**

**4 Sing praise to the Lord, You saints of His, And give
thanks at the remembrance of His holy name.**

**5 For His anger is but for a moment, His favor is for life;
Weeping may endure for a night,
But joy comes in the morning.**

. . . . .

**11 You have turned for me my mourning into dancing; You
have put off my sackcloth and clothed me with gladness,
12 To
the end that my glory may sing praise to You and not be
silent. O Lord my God, I will give thanks to You forever.**

## ***Psalm 36:7-10*** [NKJV]

**7 How precious is Your lovingkindness, O God! Therefore the
children of men put their trust under the shadow of Your wings.**

**8 They are abundantly satisfied with the fullness of Your house,
And You give them drink from the river of Your pleasures.**

**9 For with You is the fountain of life; In Your light we see light.**

**10 Oh, continue Your lovingkindness to those who know You,
And Your righteousness to the upright in heart.**

## ***Isaiah 40:11*** [RSV]

**11 He will feed his flock like a shepherd, he will gather the
lambs in his arms, he will carry them in his bosom, and
gently lead those that are with young.**

## ***Psalm 40*** [*portions*, RSV]

**[1] I waited patiently for the LORD; he inclined to me and heard my**
**cry. [2] He drew me up from the desolate pit, out of the miry**
**bog, and set my feet upon a rock, making my steps secure.**
**[3] He put a new song in my mouth, a song of praise to our God.**
**Many will see and fear, and put their trust in the LORD.**

**[4] Blessed is the man who makes the LORD his trust, who does not turn to the proud, to those who go astray after false gods!**

**[5] Thou hast multiplied, O LORD my God, thy wondrous deeds and thy thoughts toward us; none can compare with thee! Were I to proclaim and tell of them, they would be more than can be numbered.**

. . . . .

**[16] But may all who seek thee rejoice and be glad in thee; may those who love thy salvation say continually, "Great is the LORD!"**

**[17] As for me, I am poor and needy; but the Lord takes thought for me. Thou art my help and my deliverer; do not tarry, O my God!**

## ***Psalm 41:1-3*** [NKJV]

**[1] Blessed is he who considers the poor; The Lord will deliver him in**
**time of trouble. [2] The Lord will preserve him and keep him**
**alive, And he will be blessed on the earth; You will not deliver**
**him to the will of his enemies. [3] The Lord will strengthen him**
**on his bed of illness; You will sustain him on his sickbed.**

"Let the message of Christ dwell among you richly as you teach and admonish one another with all wisdom through psalms, hymns, and songs from the Spirit, singing to God with gratitude in your hearts." Colossians 3:16 [NIV]

## ***Psalm 56*** [*portions*, RSV]

**3 When I am afraid, I put my trust in thee. 4 In God, whose word I**
**praise, in God I trust without a fear. What can flesh do to me?**

**. . . . .**

**8 Thou hast kept count of my tossings; put thou my tears**
**in thy bottle! Are they not in thy book?**

**9 Then my enemies will be turned back in the day when I call.**
**This I know, that God is for me. 10 In God, whose word I praise,**
**in the LORD, whose word I praise, 11 in God I trust without a fear.**
**What can man do to me?**

## ***Psalm 63:1-8*** [NIV]

**1 You, God, are my God, earnestly I seek you; I thirst for you, my**
**whole being longs for you, in a dry and parched land where**
**there is no water. 2 I have seen you in the sanctuary and**
**beheld your power and your glory.**

**3 Because your love is better than life, my lips will glorify you.**
**4 I will praise you as long as I live, and in your name I will**
**lift up my hands.**

**5 I will be fully satisfied as with the richest of foods; with singing**
**lips my mouth will praise you. 6 On my bed I remember you;**
**I think of you through the watches of the night.**

**7 Because you are my help, I sing in the shadow of your wings.**
**8 I cling to you; your right hand upholds me.**

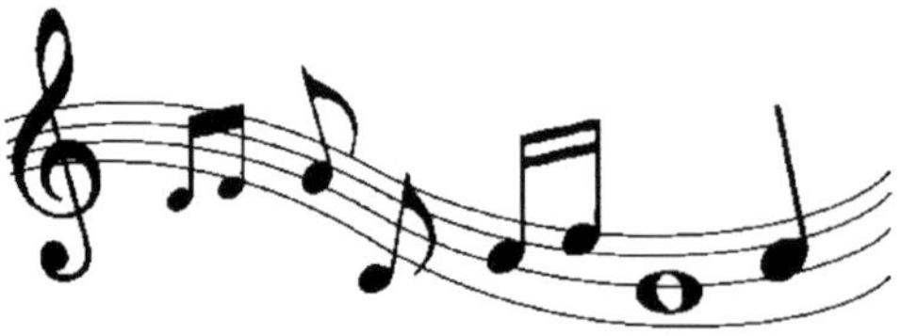

## ***Psalm 66*** [*portions*, NIV]

**[1] Shout for joy to God, all the earth! [2] Sing the glory of his name;
make his praise glorious. [3] Say to God, "How awesome are
your deeds! So great is your power that your enemies cringe
before you. [4] All the earth bows down to you; they sing
praise to you, they sing the praises of your name."**

**[5] Come and see what God has done, his awesome deeds for
mankind! [6] He turned the sea into dry land, they passed
through the waters on foot—come, let us rejoice in him.
[7] He rules forever by his power, his eyes watch the nations—
let not the rebellious rise up against him. [8] Praise our God,
all peoples, let the sound of his praise be heard; [9] he has
preserved our lives and kept our feet from slipping.**

. . . . .

**[16] Come and hear, all you who fear God; let me tell you what he
has done for me. [17] I cried out to him with my mouth; his
praise was on my tongue. [18] If I had cherished sin in my
heart, the Lord would not have listened; [19] but God has
surely listened and has heard my prayer.**

**[20] Praise be to God, who has not rejected my prayer or
withheld his love from me!**

## ***Numbers 6:24-26*** [KJV]

**[24] The LORD bless thee, and keep thee: [25] The LORD make his face
shine upon thee, and be gracious unto thee: [26] The LORD lift up his
countenance upon thee, and give thee peace.**

## ***Ephesians 1:3-4*** [NIV]

**[3] Praise be to the God and Father of our Lord Jesus Christ,
who has blessed us in the heavenly realms with every spiritual
blessing in Christ. [4] For he chose us in him before the
creation of the world to be holy and blameless in his sight.**

"Be strong. Take courage. Don't be intimidated. Don't give them a second thought because God, your God, is striding ahead of you. He's right there with you. He won't let you down; he won't leave you." Deuteronomy 31:6 [MSG]

## ***Psalm 68*** [*portions*, NIV]

**1 May God arise, may his enemies be scattered; may his foes flee**
**before him. 2 May you blow them away like smoke—as wax**
**melts before the fire, may the wicked perish before God.**

**3 But may the righteous be glad and rejoice before God; may they**
**be happy and joyful. 4 Sing to God, sing in praise of his**
**name, extol him who rides on the clouds; rejoice before**
**him—his name is the LORD.**

**5 A father to the fatherless, a defender of widows, is God in his holy**
**dwelling. 6 God sets the lonely in families, he leads out the**
**prisoners with singing; but the rebellious live in a sun-**
**scorched land.**

. . . . .

**35 You, God, are awesome in your sanctuary; the God of Israel**
**gives power and strength to his people. Praise be to God!**

## ***Psalm 73:23-28*** [NKJV]

**23 Nevertheless I am continually with You; You hold me by my**
**right hand. 24 You will guide me with Your counsel,**
**And afterward receive me to glory.**

**25 Whom have I in heaven but You? And there is none upon earth**
**that I desire besides You. 26 My flesh and my heart fail;**
**But God is the strength of my heart and my portion forever.**

**27 For indeed, those who are far from You shall perish; You have**
**destroyed all those who desert You for harlotry.**

**28 But it is good for me to draw near to God; I have put my trust**
**in the Lord God, That I may declare all Your works.**

## ***Psalm 91*** [RSV]

**[1] He who dwells in the shelter of the Most High, who abides in the**
**shadow of the Almighty, [2] will say to the LORD, "My refuge**
**and my fortress; my God, in whom I trust."**

**[3] For he will deliver you from the snare of the fowler and from the**
**deadly pestilence; [4] he will cover you with his pinions, and**
**under his wings you will find refuge; his faithfulness is a shield**
**and buckler.**

**[5] You will not fear the terror of the night, nor the arrow that flies by**
**day, [6] nor the pestilence that stalks in darkness, nor the**
**destruction that wastes at noonday.**

**[7] A thousand may fall at your side, ten thousand at your right hand;**
**but it will not come near you. [8] You will only look with your**
**eyes and see the recompense of the wicked.**

**[9] Because you have made the LORD your refuge, the Most High your**
**habitation, [10] no evil shall befall you, no scourge come near**
**your tent. [11] For he will give his angels charge of you to guard**
**you in all your ways. [12] On their hands they will bear you up,**
**lest you dash your foot against a stone.**

**[13] You will tread on the lion and the adder, the young lion and the**
**serpent you will trample under foot. [14] Because he cleaves to**
**me in love, I will deliver him; I will protect him, because he**
**knows my name. [15] When he calls to me, I will answer him; I**
**will be with him in trouble, I will rescue him and honor him.**

**[16] With long life I will satisfy him, and show him my salvation.**

## ***Isaiah 51:11-13a*** [KJV]

**[11] Therefore the redeemed of the LORD shall return, and come**
**with singing unto Zion; and everlasting joy shall be upon their**
**head: they shall obtain gladness and joy; and sorrow and**
**mourning shall flee away. [12] I, even I, am he that comforteth you:**
**who art thou, that thou shouldest be afraid of a man that shall die,**
**and of the son of man which shall be made as grass;**
**[13] And forgettest the LORD thy maker….**

***Psalm 92*** [*portions*, NKJV]

**1 It is good to give thanks to the Lord, And to sing praises to Your**
**name, O Most High; 2 To declare Your lovingkindness in the**
**morning, And Your faithfulness every night, 3 On an**
**instrument of ten strings, On the lute, And on the harp,**
**With harmonious sound.**

**4 For You, Lord, have made me glad through Your work; I will**
**triumph in the works of Your hands. 5 O Lord, how great**
**are Your works! Your thoughts are very deep.**

. . . . .

**13 Those who are planted in the house of the Lord shall flourish in the**
**courts of our God. 14 They shall still bear fruit in old age; They**
**shall be fresh and flourishing, 15 To declare that the Lord is**
**upright; He is my rock, and there is no unrighteousness in Him.**

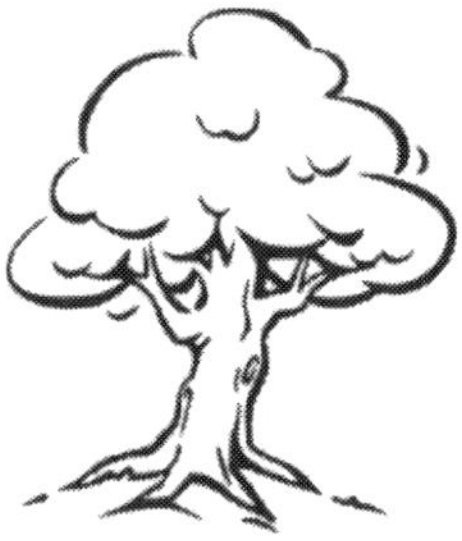

***Psalm 94:17-19*** [NKJV]

**17 Unless the Lord had been my help, My soul**
**would soon have settled in silence. 18 If I say, "My**
**foot slips," Your mercy, O Lord, will hold me up.**
**19 In the multitude of my anxieties within me,**
**Your comforts delight my soul.**

***Psalm 105:1-7*** [NKJV]

**1 Oh, give thanks to the Lord! Call upon His name; Make known His**
**deeds among the peoples! 2 Sing to Him, sing psalms to Him;**
**Talk of all His wondrous works! 3 Glory in His holy name;**
**Let the hearts of those rejoice who seek the Lord!**

**4 Seek the Lord and His strength; Seek His face evermore!**

**5 Remember His marvelous works which He has done, His wonders,**
**and the judgments of His mouth, 6 O seed of Abraham His**
**servant, You children of Jacob, His chosen ones! 7 He is the**
**Lord our God; His judgments are in all the earth.**

## ***Psalm 108*** [*portions*, NKJV]

**1 O God, my heart is steadfast; I will sing and give praise, even with
my glory. 2 Awake, lute and harp! I will awaken the dawn.
3 I will praise You, O Lord, among the peoples, And I will sing
praises to You among the nations.**

**4 For Your mercy is great above the heavens, And Your truth reaches
to the clouds. 5 Be exalted, O God, above the heavens, And
Your glory above all the earth; 6 That Your beloved may be
delivered, Save with Your right hand, and hear me.**

. . . . .

**12 Give us help from trouble, For the help of man is useless.
13 Through God we will do valiantly, For it is He who shall
tread down our enemies.**

## ***Psalm 111*** [RSV]

**1 Praise the LORD. I will give thanks to the LORD with my whole
heart, in the company of the upright, in the congregation. 2 Great
are the works of the LORD, studied by all who have pleasure in
them. 3 Full of honor and majesty is his work, and his righteousness
endures for ever. 4 He has caused his wonderful works to be
remembered; the LORD is gracious and merciful.**

**5 He provides food for those who fear him; he is ever mindful of his
covenant. 6 He has shown his people the power of his works,
in giving them the heritage of the nations.**

**7 The works of his hands are faithful and just; all his precepts are
trustworthy, 8 they are established for ever and ever,
to be performed with faithfulness and uprightness.**

**9 He sent redemption to his people; he has commanded his
covenant for ever. Holy and terrible is his name!**

**10 The fear of the LORD is the beginning of wisdom;
a good understanding have all those who practice it.
His praise endures for ever!**

## ***Psalm 107:1-32*** [NKJV]

**1 Oh, give thanks to the Lord, for He is good! For His mercy endures**
**forever.**

**2 Let the redeemed of the Lord say so, Whom He has redeemed from**
**the hand of the enemy, 3 And gathered out of the lands, From**
**the east and from the west, From the north and from the south.**

**4 They wandered in the wilderness in a desolate way; They found no**
**city to dwell in. 5 Hungry and thirsty, Their soul fainted in**
**them. 6 Then they cried out to the Lord in their trouble, And**
**He delivered them out of their distresses. 7 And He led them**
**forth by the right way, That they might go to a city for a**
**dwelling place.**

**8 Oh, that men would give thanks to the Lord for His goodness,**
**And for His wonderful works to the children of men!**
**9 For He satisfies the longing soul, And fills the hungry**
**soul with goodness.**

**10 Those who sat in darkness and in the shadow of death, Bound in**
**affliction and irons—11 Because they rebelled against the words**
**of God, And despised the counsel of the Most High,**
**12 Therefore He brought down their heart with labor; They**
**fell down, and there was none to help. 13 Then they cried out**
**to the Lord in their trouble, And He saved them out of their**
**distresses. 14 He brought them out of darkness and the**
**shadow of death, And broke their chains in pieces.**

**15 Oh, that men would give thanks to the Lord for His goodness, And**
**for His wonderful works to the children of men! 16 For He has**
**broken the gates of bronze, And cut the bars of iron in two.**

**17 Fools, because of their transgression, And because of their**
**iniquities, were afflicted. 18 Their soul abhorred all manner of**
**food, And they drew near to the gates of death. 19 Then they**
**cried out to the Lord in their trouble, And He saved them out**
**of their distresses. 20 He sent His word and healed them, And**
**delivered them from their destructions.**

[21] **Oh, that men would give thanks to the Lord for His goodness, And
for His wonderful works to the children of men! [22] Let them
sacrifice the sacrifices of thanksgiving, And declare His works
with rejoicing.**

[23] **Those who go down to the sea in ships, Who do business on great
waters, [24] They see the works of the Lord, And His wonders in
the deep. [25] For He commands and raises the stormy wind,
Which lifts up the waves of the sea. [26] They mount up to the
heavens, They go down again to the depths; Their soul melts
because of trouble. [27] They reel to and fro, and stagger like a
drunken man, And are at their wits' end. [28] Then they cry out
to the Lord in their trouble, And He brings them out of their
distresses. [29] He calms the storm, So that its waves are still.
[30] Then they are glad because they are quiet; So He guides them
to their desired haven.**

[31] **Oh, that men would give thanks to the Lord for His goodness,
And for His wonderful works to the children of men! [32] Let
them exalt Him also in the assembly of the people, And praise
Him in the company of the elders.**

## ***Psalm 112:1-8*** [KJV]

[1] **Praise ye the LORD. Blessed is the man that feareth the LORD, that
delighteth greatly in his commandments. [2] His seed shall be
mighty upon earth: the generation of the upright shall be
blessed. [3] Wealth and riches shall be in his house: and his
righteousness endureth for ever.**

[4] **Unto the upright there ariseth light in the darkness: he is gracious,
and full of compassion, and righteous.**

[5] **A good man sheweth favour, and lendeth: he will guide his affairs
with discretion. [6] Surely he shall not be moved for ever: the
righteous shall be in everlasting remembrance. [7] He shall not
be afraid of evil tidings: his heart is fixed, trusting in the
LORD.**

[8] **His heart is established, he shall not be afraid, until he see his desire
upon his enemies.**

## ***Psalm 118:24-29*** [KJV]

**24 This is the day which the LORD hath made; we will rejoice**
**and be glad in it. 25 Save now, I beseech thee, O LORD:**
**O LORD, I beseech thee, send now prosperity.**

**26 Blessed be he that cometh in the name of the LORD: we have blessed you out of the house of the LORD.**

**27 God is the LORD, which hath shewed us light: bind the sacrifice with cords, even unto the horns of the altar.**

**28 Thou art my God, and I will praise thee: thou art my God, I will exalt thee.**

**29 O give thanks unto the LORD; for he is good: for his mercy endureth for ever.**

## ***Psalm* 138** [KJV]

**1 I will praise thee with my whole heart: before the gods will I sing praise unto thee.**

**2 I will worship toward thy holy temple, and praise thy name for thy**
**lovingkindness and for thy truth: for thou hast magnified thy**
**word above all thy name. 3 In the day when I cried thou**
**answeredst me, and strengthenedst me with strength in my**
**soul.**

**4 All the kings of the earth shall praise thee, O LORD, when they**
**hear the words of thy mouth. 5 Yea, they shall sing in the ways**
**of the LORD: for great is the glory of the LORD.**

**6 Though the LORD be high, yet hath he respect unto the lowly: but the proud he knoweth afar off.**

**7 Though I walk in the midst of trouble, thou wilt revive me: thou shalt stretch forth thine hand against the wrath of mine enemies, and thy right hand shall save me.**

**8 The LORD will perfect that which concerneth me: thy mercy, O LORD, endureth for ever: forsake not the works of thine own hands.**

## ***Romans 8:31, 32, 35, 37-39*** [RSV]

**31 What then shall we say to this? If God is for us, who is against us?**
**32 He who did not spare his own Son but gave him up for us all, will he not also give us all things with him?**

. . . . .

**35 Who shall separate us from the love of Christ? Shall tribulation, or distress, or persecution, or famine, or nakedness, or peril, or sword?**

. . . . .

**37 No, in all these things we are more than conquerors through him**
**who loved us. 38 For I am sure that neither death, nor life, nor**
**angels, nor principalities, nor things present, nor things to**
**come, nor powers, 39 nor height, nor depth, nor anything else in**
**all creation, will be able to separate us from the love of God in Christ Jesus our Lord. No, in all these things we are more than conquerors through him who loved us.**

## ***Psalm 147:1-7*** [RSV]

**1 Praise the LORD! For it is good to sing praises to our God;**
**for he is gracious, and a song of praise is seemly. 2 The LORD**
**builds up Jerusalem; he gathers the outcasts of Israel.**

**3 He heals the brokenhearted, and binds up their wounds.**

**4 He determines the number of the stars,**
**he gives to all of them their names.**

**5 Great is our LORD, and abundant in power;**
**his understanding is beyond measure.**

**6 The LORD lifts up the downtrodden,**
**he casts the wicked to the ground.**

**7 Sing to the LORD with thanksgiving;**
**make melody to our God upon the lyre!**

## *Psalm 148* [NIV]

**1 Praise the LORD. Praise the LORD from the heavens;**
**praise him in the heights above.**

**2 Praise him, all his angels; praise him, all his heavenly hosts.**
**3 Praise him, sun and moon; praise him, all you shining stars.**
**4 Praise him, you highest heavens and you waters above the**
**skies.**

**5 Let them praise the name of the LORD, for at his command they**
**were created,**
**6 and he established them for ever and ever—**
**he issued a decree that will never pass away.**

**7 Praise the LORD from the earth, you great sea creatures and all**
**ocean depths,**
**8 lightning and hail, snow and clouds, stormy**
**winds that do his bidding,**
**9 you mountains and all hills,**
**fruit trees and all cedars,**
**10 wild animals and all cattle,**
**small creatures and flying birds,**
**11 kings of the earth and all**
**nations, you princes and all rulers on earth,**
**12 young men**
**and women, old men and children.**

**13 Let them praise the name of the LORD, for his name alone is**
**exalted; his splendor is above the earth and the heavens.**

**14 And he has raised up for his people a horn, the praise of all his**
**faithful servants, of Israel, the people close to his heart.**
**Praise the LORD.**

## *Revelation 4:9-11* [RSV]

**9 And whenever the living creatures give glory and honor and thanks**
**to him who is seated on the throne, who lives for ever and ever,**
**10 the twenty-four elders fall down before him who is seated on the**
**throne and worship him who lives for ever and ever;**
**they cast their crowns before the throne, singing,**

**11 "Worthy art thou, our Lord and God, to receive glory**
**and honor and power, for thou didst create all things,**
**and by thy will they existed and were created."**

# Amazing Grace!

**Amazing grace! How sweet the sound!**
**That saved a wretch like me!**
**I once was lost, but now am found,**
**Was blind, but now I see.**

**'Twas grace that taught my heart to fear,**
**And grace my fears relieved;**
**How precious did that grace appear,**
**The hour I first believed!**

**Thro' many dangers, toils and snares,**
**I have already come;**
**'Tis grace has brought me safe thus far,**
**And grace will lead me home.**

**The Lord has promised good to me,**
**His word my hope secures;**
**He will my shield and portion be,**
**As long as life endures.**

**When this flesh and heart shall fail,**
**And mortal life shall cease;**
**I shall possess, within the veil,**
**A life of joy and peace.**

**The earth shall soon dissolve like snow,**
**The sun forbear to shine;**
**But God, who called me here below,**
**Will be forever mine.** John Newton

John Newton's godly mother poured the Word of God into him until the day she died. For years he struggled between wanting to live a good life and giving himself to sin. In the servicc of the British Navy, he traveled the seas vacillating between murder and suicide. On March 10, 1748 he was in a brutal storm and cried to the Lord. He later wrote, "that tenth of March is a day much remembered by me; and I have never suffered it to pass unnoticed since the year 1748—the Lord came from on high and delivered me out of deep waters."

# Rock of Ages

**Rock of Ages, cleft for me,**
**let me hide myself in Thee.**
**Let the water and the blood,**
**from Thy wounded side which flowed,**
**be of sin the double cure;**
**save from wrath and make me pure.**

**Not the labor of my hands**
**can fulfill Thy law's demands.**
**Could my zeal no respite know,**
**could my tears forever flow?**
**All for sin could not atone;**
**Thou must save, and Thou alone.**

**Nothing in my hand I bring,**
**simply to the cross I cling.**
**Naked, come to Thee for dress;**
**helpless look to Thee for grace;**
**foul, I to the fountain fly;**
**wash me, Savior, or I die.**

**While I draw this fleeting breath,**
**when mine eyes shall close in death,**
**when I soar to worlds unknown,**
**see Thee on Thy judgment throne,**
**Rock of Ages, cleft for me,**
**let me hide myself in Thee.**

By Augustus Toplady – 1776

Sir William Wills, in a letter to Dean Lefroy, published in the [London] *Times*, says 'Toplady was one day overtaken by a thunderstorm in Burrington Comb, on the edge of my property, Blagdon, a rocky glen running up into the heart of the Mendip range, and there, taking shelter between two massive piers of our native limestone rock, he wrote, *Rock of Ages*.."

# I Need You

***"Some trust in chariots, and some in horses: but we will remember the name of the LORD our God."*** Psalm 20:7 [KJV]

**_Psalm 3:1-5_** [RSV]

**[1] O LORD, how many are my foes! Many are rising against me;**
**[2] many are saying of me, there is no help for him in God.**
**[Selah]**

**[3] But thou, O LORD, art a shield about me, my glory, and the**
**lifter of my head. [4] I cry aloud to the LORD, and he answers**
**me from his holy hill. [Selah]**

**[5] I lie down and sleep; I wake again, for the LORD sustains me.**

**_Psalm 5_** [*portions*, RSV]

**[1] Give ear to my words, O LORD; give heed to my groaning.**
**[2] Hearken to the sound of my cry, my King and my God,**
**for to thee do I pray.**

**[3] O LORD, in the morning thou dost hear my voice;**
**in the morning I prepare a sacrifice for thee, and watch.**

. . . . .

**[11] But let all who take refuge in thee rejoice, let them ever**
**sing for joy; and do thou defend them, that those who love**
**thy name may exult in thee. [12] For thou dost bless the righteous,**
**O LORD; thou dost cover him with favor as with a shield.**

***Psalm 6:2-4*** [NKJV]

**2 Have mercy on me, O Lord, for I am weak; O Lord,
heal me, for my bones are troubled. 3 My soul also is
greatly troubled; But You, O Lord—how long?**

**4 Return, O Lord, deliver me! Oh, save me for Your
mercies' sake!**

***Psalm 7:17*** [NKJV]

**17 I will praise the Lord according to His
righteousness, And will sing praise to the
name of the Lord Most High.**

***Psalm 10:12, 17, 18*** [NKJV]

**12 Arise, O Lord! O God, lift up Your hand!
Do not forget the humble.**

. . . . .

**17 Lord, You have heard the desire of the humble;
You will prepare their heart; You will cause Your
ear to hear, 18 To do justice to the fatherless and
the oppressed, That the man of the earth may
oppress no more.**

***Psalm 13:5-6*** [NKJV]

**5 But I have trusted in Your mercy;
My heart shall rejoice in Your
salvation. 6 I will sing to the Lord,
Because He has dealt bountifully
with me.**

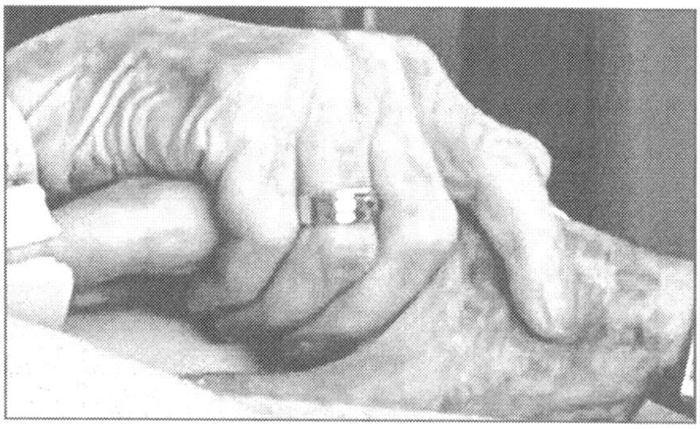

## ***Psalm 16*** [MSG]

**[1] Keep me safe, O God, I've run for dear life to you. [2] I say to**
**God, "Be my Lord!" Without you, nothing makes sense.**

**[3] And these God—God chosen lives all around—what splendid**
**friends they make!**

**[4] Don't just go shopping for a god. Gods are not for sale. I**
**swear I'll never treat god-names like brand-names. [5] My**
**choice is you, God, first and only. And now I find I'm**
**your choice! [6] You set me up with a house and yard. And**
**then you made me your heir!**

**[7] The wise counsel God gives when I'm awake is confirmed by**
**my sleeping heart. [8] Day and night I'll stick with God;**
**I've got a good thing going and I'm not letting go.**

**[9] I'm happy from the inside out, and from the outside in, I'm**
**firmly formed.**

**[10] You canceled my ticket to hell—that's not my destination!**

**[11] Now you've got my feet on the life path, all radiant from the**
**shining of your face. Ever since you took my hand, I'm**
**on the right way.**

## ***Psalm 17:6-9*** [NIV]

**[6] I call on you, my God, for you will answer me;**
**turn your ear to me and hear my prayer. [7] Show**
**me the wonders of your great love, you who save**
**by your right hand those who take refuge in you**
**from their foes.**

**[8] Keep me as the apple of your eye; hide me in the**
**shadow of your wings [9] from the wicked who are**
**out to destroy me, from my mortal enemies who**
**surround me.**

"But the Counselor, the Holy Spirit, whom the Father will send in my name, he will teach you all things, and bring to your remembrance all that I have said to you.
Peace I leave with you; my peace I give to you; not as the world gives do I give to you. Let not your hearts be troubled, neither let them be afraid." John 14:26-27 [RSV]

***Psalm 28:6-9*** [KJV]

**6 Blessed be the LORD, because he hath heard the voice of my supplications.**

**7 The LORD is my strength and my shield; my heart trusted in him, and I am helped: therefore my heart greatly rejoiceth; and with my song will I praise him.**

**8 The LORD is their strength, and he is the saving strength of his anointed.**

**9 Save thy people, and bless thine inheritance: feed them also, and lift them up for ever.**

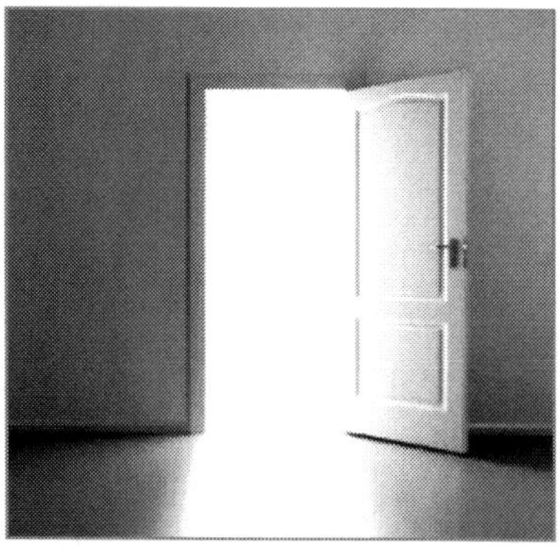

"Ask and it will be given you; seek, and you will find; knock and it will be opened to you. For every one who asks, receives; and he who seeks, finds; and to him who knocks it will be opened." Matthew 7:7-8 [RSV]

## ***Psalm 25:4-18*** [RSV]

**4 Make me to know thy ways, O LORD; teach me thy paths. 5 Lead**
**me in thy truth, and teach me, for thou art the God of my**
**salvation; for thee I wait all the day long.**

**6 Be mindful of thy mercy, O LORD, and of thy steadfast love, for**
**they have been from of old. 7 Remember not the sins of my**
**youth, or my transgressions; according to thy steadfast love**
**remember me, for thy goodness' sake, O LORD!**

**8 Good and upright is the LORD; therefore he instructs sinners in**
**the way. 9 He leads the humble in what is right, and teaches**
**the humble his way. 10 All the paths of the LORD are steadfast**
**love and faithfulness, for those who keep his covenant and his**
**testimonies.**

**11 For thy name's sake, O LORD, pardon my guilt, for it is great.**

**12 Who is the man that fears the LORD? Him will he instruct in the**
**way that he should choose. 13 He himself shall abide in**
**prosperity, and his children shall possess the land.**

**14 The friendship of the LORD is for those who fear him, and he**
**makes known to them his covenant.**

**15 My eyes are ever toward the LORD, for he will pluck my feet**
**out of the net.**

**16 Turn thou to me, and be gracious to me; for I am lonely and**
**afflicted. 17 Relieve the troubles of my heart, and bring**
**me out of my distresses.**

**18 Consider my affliction and my trouble, and forgive all my sins.**

NOTE: An **enemy** or **foe** is a relative term for any entity that's seen as forcefully adverse or threatening. It describes one who feels hatred toward, intends injury to, or opposes the interests of another. An "enemy" may also be conceptual; used to describe impersonal phenomena such as disease and a host of other things.

**Psalm 31** [*portions*, NIV]

**1 In you, LORD, I have taken refuge; let me never be put to shame;
deliver me in your righteousness.**

**2 Turn your ear to me, come quickly to my rescue; be my rock of
refuge, a strong fortress to save me. 3 Since you are my rock
and my fortress, for the sake of your name lead and guide me.**

**4 Keep me free from the trap that is set for me, for you are my refuge.
5 Into your hands I commit my spirit; deliver me, LORD, my
faithful God.**

. . . . .

**9 Be merciful to me, LORD, for I am in distress; my eyes grow weak
with sorrow, my soul and body with grief. 10 My life is
consumed by anguish and my years by groaning; my strength
fails because of my affliction, and my bones grow weak.**

. . . . .

**14 But I trust in you, LORD; I say, "You are my God." 15 My times
are in your hands; deliver me from the hands of my enemies,
from those who pursue me. 16 Let your face shine on your
servant; save me in your unfailing love.**

. . . . .

**19 How abundant are the good things that you have stored up for
those who fear you, that you bestow in the sight of all, on those
who take refuge in you. 20 In the shelter of your presence you
hide them from all human intrigues; you keep them safe in
your dwelling from accusing tongues.**

**21 Praise be to the LORD, for he showed me the wonders of his love
when I was in a city under siege.**

**22 In my alarm I said, "I am cut off from your sight!" Yet you heard
my cry for mercy when I called to you for help.**

**23 Love the LORD, all his faithful people! The LORD preserves those
who are true to him, but the proud he pays back in full.**

**24 Be strong and take heart, all you who hope in the LORD.**

## ***Psalm 39:4-12*** [NIV]

**4 "Show me, LORD, my life's end and the number of my days; let me know how fleeting my life is.**

**5 "You have made my days a mere handbreadth; the span of my years is as nothing before you. Everyone is but a breath, even those who seem secure.**

**6 "Surely everyone goes around like a mere phantom; in vain they rush about, heaping up wealth without knowing whose it will finally be.**

**7 "But now, Lord, what do I look for? My hope is in you. 8 Save me**
**from all my transgressions; do not make me the scorn of fools.**

**9 "I was silent; I would not open my mouth, for you are the one who**
**has done this. 10 Remove your scourge from me; I am**
**overcome by the blow of your hand. 11 When you rebuke and**
**discipline anyone for their sin, you consume their wealth like a moth—surely everyone is but a breath.**

**12 "Hear my prayer, LORD, listen to my cry for help; do not be deaf to my weeping. I dwell with you as a foreigner, a stranger, as all my ancestors were. …."**

## ***Psalm 54*** [NIV]

**1 Save me, O God, by your name; vindicate me by your might.**
**2 Hear my prayer, O God; listen to the words of my mouth.**
**3 Arrogant foes are attacking me; ruthless people are trying to kill me—people without regard for God.**

**4 Surely God is my help; the Lord is the one who sustains me.**
**5 Let evil recoil on those who slander me;**
**in your faithfulness destroy them.**

**6 I will sacrifice a freewill offering to you; I will praise your**
**name, LORD, for it is good. 7 You have delivered me from all**
**my troubles, and my eyes have looked in triumph on my foes.**

## *Psalm 61:1-4* [KJV]

**1 Hear my cry, O God; attend unto my prayer.**

**2 From the end of the earth will I cry unto thee,
when my heart is overwhelmed: lead me to the
rock that is higher than I. 3 For thou hast been a
shelter for me, and a strong tower from the enemy.**

**4 I will abide in thy tabernacle for ever: I will trust
in the covert of thy wings. Selah.**

## *Psalm 55* [*portions*, NKJV]

**1 Give ear to my prayer, O God, And do not hide Yourself from my
supplication. 2 Attend to me, and hear me; I am restless in my
complaint, and moan noisily, 3 Because of the voice of the
enemy, Because of the oppression of the wicked; For they bring
down trouble upon me, And in wrath they hate me.**

**4 My heart is severely pained within me, And the terrors of death
have fallen upon me. 5 Fearfulness and trembling have come
upon me, And horror has overwhelmed me.**

**6 So I said, "Oh, that I had wings like a dove! I would fly away and be
at rest. 7 Indeed, I would wander far off, And remain in the
wilderness. Selah. 8 I would hasten my escape From the windy
storm and tempest."**

. . . . .

**16 As for me, I will call upon God, And the Lord shall save me.
17 Evening and morning and at noon I will pray, and cry aloud,
And He shall hear my voice. 18 He has redeemed my soul in
peace from the battle that was against me ....**

And Jesus said to him, "If you can! All things are possible to him who believes."

Immediately the father of the child cried out and said, "I believe; help my unbelief!" Mark 9:23-24 [RSV]

## *Psalm 57:7-11* [NIV]

**7 My heart, O God, is steadfast, my heart is steadfast; I will sing and make music.**

**8 Awake, my soul! Awake, harp and lyre! I will awaken the dawn.**

**9 I will praise you, Lord, among the nations; I will**
**sing of you among the peoples. 10 For great is**
**your love, reaching to the heavens; your faithfulness reaches to the skies.**

**11 Be exalted, O God, above the heavens; let your glory be over all the earth.**

## *Psalm 62:5-12* [NIV]

**5 Yes, my soul, find rest in God; my hope comes from him. 6 Truly he**
**is my rock and my salvation; he is my fortress, I will not be**
**shaken. 7 My salvation and my honor depend on God; he is**
**my mighty rock, my refuge.**

**8 Trust in him at all times, you people; pour out your hearts to him,**
**for God is our refuge. 9 Surely the lowborn are but a breath,**
**the highborn are but a lie. If weighed on a balance, they are nothing; together they are only a breath.**

**10 Do not trust in extortion or put vain hope in stolen goods; though your riches increase, do not set your heart on them.**

**11 One thing God has spoken, two things I have heard: "Power**
**belongs to you, God, 12 and with you, Lord, is unfailing love";**
**and, "You reward everyone according to what they have done."**

## *Psalm 141:1-2* [NIV]

**1 I call to you, LORD, come quickly to me; hear me when I call to**
**you. 2 May my prayer be set before you like incense; may the lifting**
**up of my hands be like the evening sacrifice.**

## ***Psalm 69*** [*portions*, NKJV]

**1 Save me, O God! For the waters have come up to my neck. 2 I sink**
**in deep mire, Where there is no standing; I have come into**
**deep waters, Where the floods overflow me.**

**3 I am weary with my crying; My throat is dry; My eyes fail while I**
**wait for my God.**

. . . . .

**13 But as for me, my prayer is to You, O Lord, in the acceptable**
**time; O God, in the multitude of Your mercy, Hear me in the**
**truth of Your salvation.**

**14 Deliver me out of the mire, And let me not sink; Let me be**
**delivered from those who hate me, And out of the deep waters.**
**15 Let not the floodwater overflow me, Nor let the deep**
**swallow me up; And let not the pit shut its mouth on me.**

**16 Hear me, O Lord, for Your lovingkindness is good; Turn to me**
**according to the multitude of Your tender mercies. 17 And do**
**not hide Your face from Your servant, For I am in trouble;**
**Hear me speedily. 18 Draw near to my soul, and redeem it;**
**Deliver me because of my enemies.**

. . . . .

**30 I will praise the name of God with a song, And will magnify Him**
**with thanksgiving. 31 This also shall please the Lord better**
**than an ox or bull, Which has horns and hooves.**

**32 The humble shall see this and be glad; And you who seek God,**
**your hearts shall live. 33 For the Lord hears the poor, And**
**does not despise His prisoners.**

**34 Let heaven and earth praise Him, The seas and everything that**
**moves in them.**

## ***Psalm 141:8*** [NIV]

**8 But my eyes are fixed on you, Sovereign LORD;**
**in you I take refuge—do not give me over to death.**

## ***Psalm 70*** [NKJV]

**[1] To bring to remembrance. Make haste, O God, to**
**deliver me! Make haste to help me, O Lord!**

**[2] Let them be ashamed and confounded**
**Who seek my life; Let them be turned back and**
**confused who desire my hurt. [3] Let them be turned**
**back because of their shame, Who say, "Aha, aha!"**

**[4] Let all those who seek You rejoice and be glad in**
**You; And let those who love Your salvation say**
**continually, "Let God be magnified!"**

**[5] But I am poor and needy; Make haste to me,**
**O God! You are my help and my deliverer;**
**O Lord, do not delay.**

## ***Psalm 77*** [*portions*, NKJV]

**[1] I cried out to God with my voice—To God with my voice; And He**
**gave ear to me. [2] In the day of my trouble I sought the Lord;**
**My hand was stretched out in the night without ceasing; My**
**soul refused to be comforted. [3] I remembered God, and was**
**troubled; I complained, and my spirit was overwhelmed. Selah**

**[4] You hold my eyelids open; I am so troubled that I cannot speak.**

**[5] I have considered the days of old, The years of ancient times. [6] I call**
**to remembrance my song in the night; I meditate within my**
**heart, And my spirit makes diligent search.**

. . . . . .

**[11] I will remember the works of the Lord; Surely I will remember**
**Your wonders of old. [12] I will also meditate on all Your work,**
**And talk of Your deeds.**

**[13] Your way, O God, is in the sanctuary; Who is so great a God as our**
**God? [14] You are the God who does wonders; You have**
**declared Your strength among the peoples.**

## *Psalm 71* [RSV]

**[1] In thee, O LORD, do I take refuge; let me never be put to shame!**

**[2] In thy righteousness deliver me and rescue me; incline thy ear to**
**me, and save me! [3] Be thou to me a rock of refuge, a strong**
**fortress, to save me, for thou art my rock and my fortress.**

**[4] Rescue me, O my God, from the hand of the wicked, from the grasp**
**of the unjust and cruel man. [5] For thou, O Lord, art my hope,**
**my trust, O LORD, from my youth. [6] Upon thee I have leaned**
**from my birth; thou art he who took me from my mother's**
**womb. My praise is continually of thee.**

**[7] I have been as a portent to many; but thou art my strong refuge.**
**[8] My mouth is filled with thy praise, and with thy glory all the**
**day.**

**[9] Do not cast me off in the time of old age; forsake me not when my**
**strength is spent. [10] For my enemies speak concerning me,**
**those who watch for my life consult together, [11] and say, "God**
**has forsaken him; pursue and seize him, for there is none to**
**deliver him."**

**[12] O God, be not far from me; O my God, make haste to help me!**
**[13] May my accusers be put to shame and consumed; with scorn**
**and disgrace may they be covered who seek my hurt.**

**[14] But I will hope continually, and will praise thee yet more and more.**
**[15] My mouth will tell of thy righteous acts, of thy deeds of**
**salvation all the day, for their number is past my knowledge.**
**[16] With the mighty deeds of the Lord GOD I will come, I will**
**praise thy righteousness, thine alone.**

**[17] O God, from my youth thou hast taught me, and I still proclaim thy**
**wondrous deeds. [18] So even to old age and gray hairs, O God,**
**do not forsake me, till I proclaim thy might to all the**
**generations to come. Thy power [19] and thy righteousness, O**
**God, reach the high heavens. Thou who hast done great things,**
**O God, who is like thee?**

20 Thou who hast made me see many sore troubles wilt revive me
again; from the depths of the earth thou wilt bring me up
again. 21 Thou wilt increase my honor, and comfort me again.

22 I will also praise thee with the harp for thy faithfulness, O my God;
I will sing praises to thee with the lyre, O Holy One of Israel.

23 My lips will shout for joy, when I sing praises to thee; my soul also,
which thou hast rescued.

24 And my tongue will talk of thy righteous help all the day long, for
they have been put to shame and disgraced who sought to do
me hurt.

## *Psalm 80:19* [NIV]

19 Restore us, LORD God Almighty;
make your face shine on us, that we may be saved.

## *Psalm 85:7-13* [NIV]

7 Show us your unfailing love, LORD,
and grant us your salvation.

8 I will listen to what God the LORD says;
he promises peace to his people,
his faithful servants—but let them
not turn to folly.

9 Surely his salvation is near those who fear him,
that his glory may dwell in our land.

10 Love and faithfulness meet together;
righteousness and peace kiss each other.

11 Faithfulness springs forth from the earth, and
righteousness looks down from heaven.

12 The LORD will indeed give what is good,
and our land will yield its harvest.

13 Righteousness goes before him and
prepares the way for his steps.

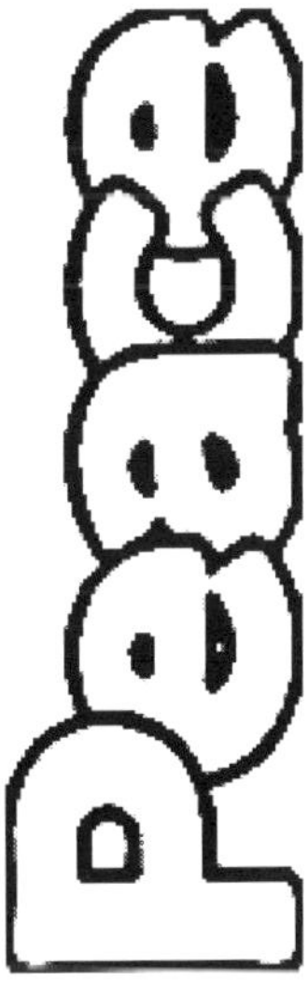

## ***Psalm 86*** [*portions*, NIV]

**1 Hear me, LORD, and answer me, for I am poor and needy.**

**2 Guard my life, for I am faithful to you; save your servant who trusts
in you. You are my God; 3 have mercy on me, Lord, for I call to
you all day long. 4 Bring joy to your servant, Lord, for I put
my trust in you.**

**5 You, Lord, are forgiving and good, abounding in love to all who call
to you. 6 Hear my prayer, LORD; listen to my cry for mercy.
7 When I am in distress, I call to you, because you answer me.**

**8 Among the gods there is none like you, Lord; no deeds can compare
with yours.**

. . . . .

**11 Teach me your way, LORD, that I may rely on your faithfulness;
give me an undivided heart, that I may fear your name.**

**12 I will praise you, Lord my God, with all my heart; I will glorify
your name forever. 13 For great is your love toward me; you
have delivered me from the depths, from the realm of the dead.**

## ***Psalm 88:1-3*** [NIV]

**1 LORD, you are the God who saves me; day and night I cry out to
you. 2 May my prayer come before you; turn your ear to my cry.
3 I am overwhelmed with troubles and my life draws near to death.**

## ***Psalm 144:1-4*** [RSV]

**1 Blessed be the LORD, my rock, who trains my hands for war,
and my fingers for battle; 2 my rock and my fortress,
my stronghold and my deliverer, my shield and
he in whom I take refuge, who subdues the
peoples under him. 3 O LORD, what is man that
thou dost regard him, or the son of man that thou
dost think of him? 4 Man is like a breath,
his days are like a passing shadow.**

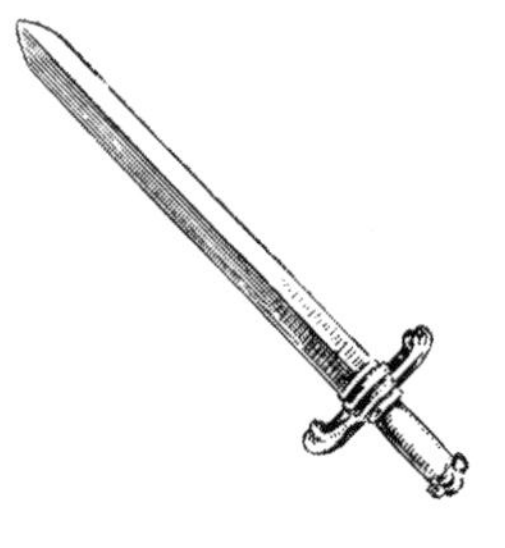

## ***Psalm 102*** [*portions*, NKJV]

**1 A Prayer of the afflicted, when he is overwhelmed and pours out his complaint before the Lord. Hear my prayer, O Lord, And let my cry come to You.**

**2 Do not hide Your face from me in the day of my trouble; Incline Your ear to me; In the day that I call, answer me speedily.**

. . . . .

**16 For the Lord shall build up Zion; He shall appear in His glory.**

**17 He shall regard the prayer of the destitute, And shall not despise their prayer.**

**18 This will be written for the generation to come, That a people yet to be created may praise the Lord.**

. . . . .

**25 Of old You laid the foundation of the earth, And the heavens are**
**the work of Your hands. 26 They will perish, but You will endure;**
**Yes, they will all grow old like a garment; Like a cloak You will**
**change them, And they will be changed.**

**27 But You are the same, And Your years will have no end.**

## ***Psalm 109:21-26*** [NIV]

**21 But you, Sovereign LORD, help me for your**
**name's sake; out of the goodness of your love,**
**deliver me. 22 For I am poor and needy, and my**
**heart is wounded within me.**

**23 I fade away like an evening shadow; I am shaken**
**off like a locust. 24 My knees give way from fasting;**
**my body is thin and gaunt. 25 I am an object of**
**scorn to my accusers; when they see me, they shake**
**their heads.**

**26 Help me, LORD my God; save me according to your unfailing love.**

## ***Psalm 119*** [*portions*, NIV]

**73 Your hands made me and formed me; give me
understanding to learn your commands. 74 May those
who fear you rejoice when they see me, for I have put
my hope in your word.**

**75 I know, LORD, that your laws are righteous, and that in
faithfulness you have afflicted me. 76 May your
unfailing love be my comfort, according to your
promise to your servant. 77 Let your compassion come
to me that I may live, for your law is my delight.**

. . . . .

**89 Your word, LORD, is eternal; it stands firm in the
heavens. 90 Your faithfulness continues through all
generations; you established the earth, and it endures.**

**91 Your laws endure to this day, for all things serve you.
92 If your law had not been my delight, I would have
perished in my affliction. 93 I will never forget your
precepts, for by them you have preserved my life.**

**94 Save me, for I am yours; I have sought out your precepts.**

. . . . .

**145 I call with all my heart; answer me, LORD, and I will
obey your decrees. 146 I call out to you; save me and I
will keep your statutes. 147 I rise before dawn and cry
for help; I have put my hope in your word.**

**148 My eyes stay open through the watches of the night,
that I may meditate on your promises.**

**149 Hear my voice in accordance with your love; preserve my
life, LORD, according to your laws.**

**150 Those who devise wicked schemes are near, but they are
far from your law. 151 Yet you are near, LORD, and all
your commands are true.**

## ***Psalm 131*** [RSV]

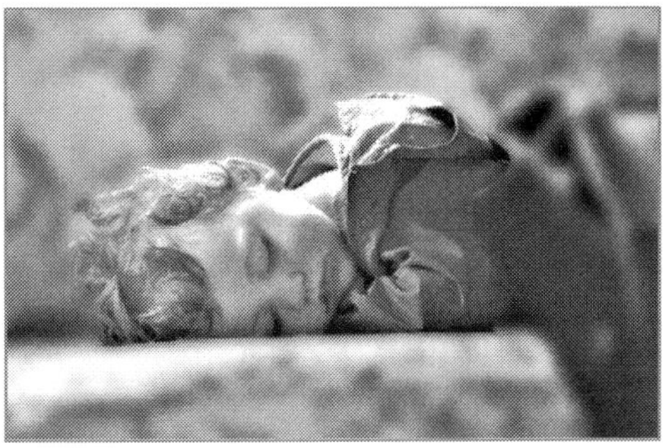

1 **O LORD, my heart is not lifted up, my eyes are not raised too high; I do not occupy myself with things too great and too marvelous for me.**

2 **But I have calmed and quieted my soul, like a child quieted at its mother's breast; like a child that is quieted is my soul.**

3 **O Israel, hope in the LORD from this time forth and for evermore.**

## ***Psalm 142:5-7*** [RSV]

5 **I cry to thee, O LORD; I say, Thou art my refuge, my portion in the land of the living.**

6 **Give heed to my cry; for I am brought very low! Deliver me from my persecutors; for they are too strong for me!**

7 **Bring me out of prison, that I may give thanks to thy name! The righteous will surround me; for thou wilt deal bountifully with me.**

For this thing I besought the Lord thrice, that it might depart from me.

And he said unto me, My grace is sufficient for thee: for my strength is made perfect in weakness. Most gladly therefore will I rather glory in my infirmities, that the power of Christ may rest upon me.

2 Corinthians 12:8-9 [KJV]

## ***Psalm 143:5-8*** [KJV]

**[5] I remember the days of old; I meditate on all thy works;**
**I muse on the work of thy hands.**

**[6] I stretch forth my hands unto thee: my soul thirsteth after**
**thee, as a thirsty land. Selah.**

**[7] Hear me speedily, O LORD: my spirit faileth: hide not thy**
**face from me, lest I be like unto them that go down**
**into the pit.**

**[8] Cause me to hear thy lovingkindness in the morning; for**
**in thee do I trust: cause me to know the way wherein**
**I should walk; for I lift up my soul unto thee.**

## ***Lamentations 3:19-26*** [RSV]

**[19] Remember my affliction and my bitterness,**
**the wormwood and the gall! [20] My soul**
**continually thinks of it and is bowed**
**down within me.**

**[21] But this I call to mind, and therefore I have**
**hope: [22] The steadfast love of the LORD**
**never ceases, his mercies never come to**
**an end; [23] they are new every morning;**
**great is thy faithfulness.**

**[24] "The LORD is my portion," says my soul,**
**"therefore I will hope in him."**

**[25] The LORD is good to those who wait for him,**
**to the soul that seeks him. [26] It is good that**
**one should wait quietly for the salvation of**
**the LORD.**

***Isaiah 49:13-16*** [RSV]

**13 Sing for joy, O heavens, and exult, O earth;**
**break forth, O mountains, into singing!**
**For the LORD has comforted his people,**
**and will have compassion on his afflicted.**

**14 But Zion said, "The LORD has forsaken me,**
**my LORD has forgotten me."**

**15 Can a woman forget her sucking child,**
**that she should have no compassion on the**
**son of her womb? Even these may forget,**
**yet I will not forget you.**

**16 Behold, I have graven you on the palms of my**
**hands; your walls are continually before me.**

***Isaiah 61:1-3*** [RSV]

**1 The Spirit of the Lord GOD is upon me, because**
**the LORD has anointed me to bring good**
**tidings to the afflicted; he has sent me to bind**
**up the brokenhearted, to proclaim liberty to**
**the captives, and the opening of the prison to**
**those who are bound;**

**2 to proclaim the year of the LORD's favor, and the**
**day of vengeance of our God; to comfort all**
**who mourn;**

**3 to grant to those who mourn in Zion—to give**
**them a garland instead of ashes, the oil of**
**gladness instead of mourning, the mantle of**
**praise instead of a faint spirit; that they may**
**be called oaks of righteousness, the planting**
**of the LORD, that he may be glorified.**

## ***Isaiah 60*** [*portions*, RSV]

**1 Arise, shine; for your light has come, and the glory of the LORD has risen upon you.**

**2 For behold, darkness shall cover the earth, and thick darkness the peoples; but the LORD will arise upon you, and his glory will**
**be seen upon you. 3 And nations shall come to your light, and**
**kings to the brightness of your rising.**

**4 Lift up your eyes round about, and see; they all gather together, they come to you; your sons shall come from far, and your daughters shall be carried in the arms.**

**5 Then you shall see and be radiant, your heart shall thrill and rejoice; because the abundance of the sea shall be turned to you, the wealth of the nations shall come to you.**

. . . . .

**15 Whereas you have been forsaken and hated, with no one passing**
**through, I will make you majestic for ever, a joy from age to**
**age. 16 You shall suck the milk of nations, you shall suck the**
**breast of kings; and you shall know that I, the LORD, am**
**your Savior and your Redeemer, the Mighty One of Jacob.**

**17 Instead of bronze I will bring gold, and instead of iron I will bring silver; instead of wood, bronze, instead of stones, iron. I will make your overseers peace and your taskmasters righteousness.**

**18 Violence shall no more be heard in your land, devastation or destruction within your borders; you shall call your walls Salvation, and your gates Praise.**

**19 The sun shall be no more your light by day, nor for brightness**
**shall the moon give light to you by night; but the LORD will**
**be your everlasting light, and your God will be your glory.**
**20 Your sun shall no more go down, nor your moon withdraw**
**itself; for the LORD will be your everlasting light, and your**
**days of mourning shall be ended.**

21 Your people shall all be righteous; they shall possess the land for
ever, the shoot of my planting, the work of my hands, that I
might be glorified. 22 The least one shall become a clan, and the
smallest one a mighty nation; I am the LORD; in its time I will
hasten it.

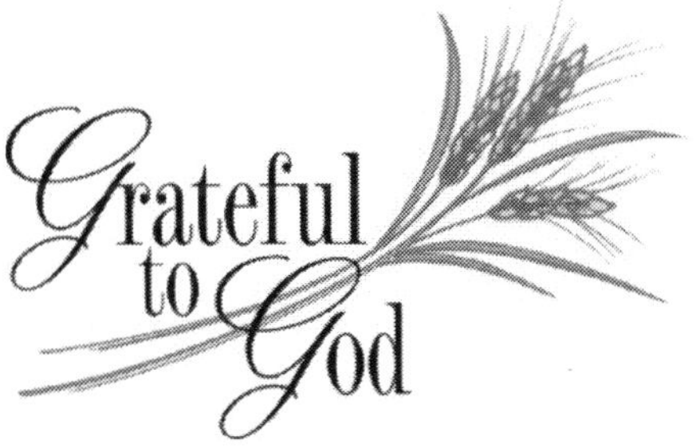


## ***Luke 4:38-44*** [NIV]

38 Jesus left the synagogue and went to the home of Simon.
Now Simon's mother-in-law was suffering from a high
fever, and they asked Jesus to help her. 39 So he bent
over her and rebuked the fever, and it left her. She got
up at once and began to wait on them.

40 At sunset, the people brought to Jesus all who had various kinds of sickness, and laying his hands on each one, he healed them.

41 Moreover, demons came out of many people, shouting, "You are the Son of God!" But he rebuked them and would not allow them to speak, because they knew he was the Messiah.

42 At daybreak, Jesus went out to a solitary place. The people were looking for him and when they came to where he was, they tried to keep him from leaving them.

43 But he said, "I must proclaim the good news of the kingdom of God to the other towns also, because that is why I was sent."

44 And he kept on preaching in the synagogues of Judea.

## *Luke 5:12-16* [NIV]

[12] **While Jesus was in one of the towns, a man came along who was covered with leprosy. When he saw Jesus, he fell with his face to the ground and begged him, "Lord, if you are willing, you can make me clean."**

[13] **Jesus reached out his hand and touched the man. "I am willing," he said. "Be clean!" And immediately the leprosy left him.**

[14] **Then Jesus ordered him, "Don't tell anyone, but go, show yourself to the priest and offer the sacrifices that Moses commanded for your cleansing, as a testimony to them."**

[15] **Yet the news about him spread all the more, so that crowds of people came to hear him and to be healed of their sicknesses.**

[16] **But Jesus often withdrew to lonely places and prayed.**

## *Luke 7:11-17* [NIV]

[11] **Soon afterward, Jesus went to a town called Nain, and his disciples and a large crowd went along with him.**

[12] **As he approached the town gate, a dead person was being carried out—the only son of his mother, and she was a widow. And a large crowd from the town was with her.**

[13] **When the Lord saw her, his heart went out to her and he said, "Don't cry."**

[14] **Then he went up and touched the bier they were carrying him on, and the bearers stood still. He said, "Young man, I say to you, get up!"**

[15] **The dead man sat up and began to talk, and Jesus gave him back to his mother.**

[16] **They were all filled with awe and praised God. "A great prophet has appeared among us," they said. "God has come to help his people."**

[17] **This news about Jesus spread throughout Judea and the surrounding country.**

## ***Luke 18:35-43*** [NIV]

**35 As Jesus approached Jericho, a blind man was sitting by the**
**roadside begging. 36 When he heard the crowd going by,**
**he asked what was happening.**

**37 They told him, "Jesus of Nazareth is passing by."**

**38 He called out, "Jesus, Son of David, have mercy on me!"**

**39 Those who led the way rebuked him and told him to be quiet, but he shouted all the more, "Son of David, have mercy on me!"**

**40 Jesus stopped and ordered the man to be brought to him. When he came near, Jesus asked him,**

**41 "What do you want me to do for you?"**

**"Lord, I want to see," he replied.**

**42 Jesus said to him, "Receive your sight; your faith has healed you."**

**43 Immediately he received his sight and followed Jesus, praising God. When all the people saw it, they also praised God.**

## ***John 11:25-26*** [KJV]

**25 Jesus said unto her, I am the resurrection, and the life:**
**he that believeth in me, though he were dead, yet shall he live:**
**26 And whosoever liveth and believeth in me shall never die.**
**Believest thou this?**

Love is patient, love is kind. It does not envy, it does not boast, it is not proud. It does not dishonor others, it is not self-seeking, it is not easily angered, it keeps no record of wrongs. Love does not delight in evil but rejoices with the truth. It always protects, always trusts, always hopes, always perseveres. Love never fails.

1 Corinthians 13:4-8a [NIV]

## ***Revelations of John 22*** [*portions*, KJV]

**[1] And he shewed me a pure river of water of life, clear as crystal,
proceeding out of the throne of God and of the Lamb. [2] In the
midst of the street of it, and on either side of the river, was
there the tree of life, which bare twelve manner of fruits, and
yielded her fruit every month: and the leaves of the tree were
for the healing of the nations.**

**[3] And there shall be no more curse: but the throne of God and of the
Lamb shall be in it; and his servants shall serve him: [4] And
they shall see his face; and his name shall be in their foreheads.
[5] And there shall be no night there; and they need no candle,
neither light of the sun; for the Lord God giveth them light:
and they shall reign for ever and ever.**

. . . . .

**[12] And, behold, I come quickly; and my reward is with me, to give
every man according as his work shall be. [13] I am Alpha and
Omega, the beginning and the end, the first and the last.**

**[14] Blessed are they that do his commandments, that they may have
right to the tree of life, and may enter in through the gates into
the city. [15] For without are dogs, and sorcerers, and
whoremongers, and murderers, and idolaters, and whosoever
loveth and maketh a lie.**

**[16] I Jesus have sent mine angel to testify unto you these things in the churches. I am the root and the offspring of David, and the bright and morning star.**

**[17] And the Spirit and the bride say, Come. And let him that heareth say, Come. And let him that is athirst come. And whosoever will, let him take the water of life freely.**

**[18] For I testify unto every man that heareth the words of the prophecy
of this book, If any man shall add unto these things, God shall
add unto him the plagues that are written in this book: [19] And
if any man shall take away from the words of the book of this
prophecy, God shall take away his part out of the book of life,
and out of the holy city, and from the things which are written
in this book.**

# What a Friend We Have in Jesus

**What a Friend we have in Jesus, all our sins and griefs to bear!
What a privilege to carry, everything to God in prayer!
Oh, what peace we often forfeit, oh what needless pain we bear.
All because we do not carry, everything to God in Prayer!**

**Have we trials and temptations? Is there trouble anywhere?
We should never be discouraged; take it to the Lord in prayer.
Can we find a friend so faithful, who will all our sorrows share?
Jesus knows our every weakness, take it to the Lord in prayer.**

**Are we weak and heavy laden, cumbered with a load of care?
Precious Savior, still our refuge! Take it to the Lord in prayer.
Do thy friends despise, forsake thee?
Take it to the Lord in prayer.
In His arms He'll take and shield Thee,
Thou wilt find a solace there.**

Lyrics by Joseph M Scriven, 1855
Music by Charles C. Converse

Joseph Scriven was born in Ireland but emigrated to Canada when he was 25 years old. Ten years later, he received word that his mother was facing a crisis. Joseph wrote this poem and sent it to her; his mother shared it with a friend and it was published anonymously in 1855.

Until a short time before his death, it was not known that he had a poetic gift. A neighbor, sitting up with him in his illness, happened upon a manuscript copy of "What a Friend We Have in Jesus." Reading it with great delight and questioning Mr. Scriven about it, he said that he had composed it for his mother, to comfort her in a time of special sorrow, not intending that anyone else should see it. Sometime later, when another Port Hope neighbor asked him if it was true that he composed the hymn, his reply was, "The Lord and I did it between us."

# The Old Rugged Cross

**On a hill far away stood an old rugged cross,**
**The emblem of suffering and shame;**
**And I love that old cross where the dearest and best**
**For a world of lost sinners was slain.**

**O that old rugged cross, so despised by the world,**
**Has a wondrous attraction for me;**
**For the dear Lamb of God left His glory above**
**To bear it to dark Calvary.**

**In that old rugged cross, stained with blood so divine,**
**A wondrous beauty I see,**
**For ’twas on that old cross Jesus suffered and died,**
**To pardon and sanctify me.**

**To the old rugged cross I will ever be true;**
**Its shame and reproach gladly bear;**
**Then He’ll call me some day to my home far away,**
**Where His glory forever I’ll share.**

**So I’ll cherish the old rugged cross,**
**Till my trophies at last I lay down;**
**I will cling to the old rugged cross,**
**And exchange it some day for a crown.**

By George Bennard

When Bennard was very young, his family moved to Albia, Iowa, then Lucas, Iowa. He wanted a career in evangelism, but was forced instead to support his mother and sisters when his father died. After marrying, he and his wife worked for the Salvation Army in Illinois, and he later served as an evangelist in America and Canada. Bennard spent his last years in Reed City, Michigan, where the Chamber of Commerce erected a cross near his home. The Old Rugged Cross Historical Museum in Reed City commemorates his work.

# Forgive Me

***"Look upon mine affliction and my pain; and forgive all my sins."***
Psalm 25:18 [KJV]

***Isaiah 53:6a*** [RSV]

**All we like sheep have gone astray;**
**we have turned every one to his own way….**

***Psalm 14:2-3*** [RSV]

**2 The LORD looks down from heaven upon the children of men, to see if there are any that act wisely, that seek after God. 3 They have all gone astray, they are all alike corrupt; there is none that does good and sins not, no not one.**

***Psalm 143:1-2*** [RSV]

**1 Hear my prayer, O LORD! Give ear to my supplications!**
**In your faithfulness answer me, in your righteousness!**

**2 Enter not into judgment with your servant;**
**for no man living is righteous before you.**

***Romans 3:23b*** [RSV]

**… All have sinned and fallen short of the glory of God.**

## ***1 John 1:8-9*** [RSV]

**8 If we say that we have no sin, we deceive ourselves, and the truth is**
**not in us. 9 If we confess our sins, he is faithful and just, and will**
**forgive our sins and cleanse us from all unrighteousness.**

## ***John 3:16-17*** [RSV]

**16 For God so loved the world that he gave his only Son, that whoever believes in him should not perish but have eternal life.**

**17 For God sent the Son into the world, not to condemn the world, but that the world might be saved through him.**

## ***Romans 5:1-5*** [RSV]

**1 Therefore, since we are justified by faith, we have peace with God through our Lord Jesus Christ.**

**2 Through him we have obtained access to this grace in which we stand, and we rejoice in our hope of sharing the glory of God.**

**3 More than that, we rejoice in our sufferings, knowing**
**that suffering produces endurance, 4 and endurance**
**produces character, and character produces hope,**
**5 and hope does not disappoint us, because God's love**
**has been poured into our hearts through the Holy**
**Spirit which has been given to us.**

## ***Romans 5:6-9*** [NIV]

**6 You see, at just the right time, when we were still powerless,**
**Christ died for the ungodly. 7 Very rarely will anyone die**
**for a righteous person, though for a good person someone**
**might possibly dare to die. 8 But God demonstrates his own**
**love for us in this: While we were still sinners, Christ died for**
**us. 9 Since we have now been justified by his blood, how much**
**more shall we be saved from God's wrath through him!**

## ***Psalm 51*** [*portions*, NKJV]

**1 Have mercy upon me, O God, According to Your lovingkindness;**
**According to the multitude of Your tender mercies,**
**Blot out my transgressions.**

**2 Wash me thoroughly from my iniquity, And cleanse me from my**
**sin. 3 For I acknowledge my transgressions, And my sin is**
**always before me. 4 Against You, You only, have I sinned,**
**And done this evil in Your sight—That You may be found**
**just when You speak, And blameless when You judge.**

. . . . .

**9 Hide Your face from my sins, And blot out all my iniquities.**
**10 Create in me a clean heart, O God, And renew a steadfast**
**spirit within me. 11 Do not cast me away from Your presence,**
**And do not take Your Holy Spirit from me. 12 Restore to me**
**the joy of Your salvation, And uphold me by Your generous**
**Spirit.**

## ***Psalm 79:8-13*** [NKJV]

**8 Oh, do not remember former iniquities against us! Let Your tender**
**mercies come speedily to meet us, For we have been brought**
**very low. 9 Help us, O God of our salvation, For the glory of**
**Your name; And deliver us, and provide atonement for our**
**sins, For Your name's sake!**

**10 Why should the nations say, "Where is their God?" Let there be**
**known among the nations in our sight the avenging of the blood**
**of Your servants which has been shed.**

**11 Let the groaning of the prisoner come before You; According to the**
**greatness of Your power preserve those who are appointed to**
**die; 12 And return to our neighbors sevenfold into their bosom**
**Their reproach with which they have reproached You, O Lord.**

**13 So we, Your people and sheep of Your pasture,**
**Will give You thanks forever; We will show forth**
**Your praise to all generations.**

## ***Psalm 130*** [NKJV]

**1 Out of the depths I have cried to You, O Lord;**
**2 Lord, hear my voice! Let Your ears be attentive**
**To the voice of my supplications.**

**3 If You, Lord, should mark iniquities, O Lord, who could stand?**
**4 But there is forgiveness with You, That You may be feared.**

**5 I wait for the Lord, my soul waits, And in His word I do hope. 6 My**
**soul waits for the Lord more than those who watch for the**
**morning—Yes, more than those who watch for the morning.**

**7 O Israel, hope in the Lord; For with the Lord there is mercy, And**
**with Him is abundant redemption. 8 And He shall redeem**
**Israel from all his iniquities.**

## ***Luke 1:26-38*** [RSV]

**26 In the sixth month the angel Gabriel was sent from God to a city**
**of Galilee named Nazareth, 27 to a virgin betrothed to a man**
**whose name was Joseph, of the house of David; and the virgin's**
**name was Mary.**

**28 And he came to her and said, "Hail, O favored one, the Lord is**
**with you!"**

**29 But she was greatly troubled at the saying, and considered in her**
**mind what sort of greeting this might be.**

**30 And the angel said to her, "Do not be afraid, Mary, for you have**
**found favor with God. 31 And behold, you will conceive in your**
**womb and bear a son, and you shall call his name Jesus. 32 He**
**will be great, and will be called the Son of the Most High; and**
**the Lord God will give to him the throne of his father David,**
**33 and he will reign over the house of Jacob for ever; and of his**
**kingdom there will be no end."**

**34 And Mary said to the angel, "How shall this be, since I have no**
**husband?"**

**35 And the angel said to her, "The Holy Spirit will come upon you,**
**and the power of the Most High will overshadow you; therefore**

**the child to be born will be called holy, the Son of God. 36 And
behold, your kinswoman Elizabeth in her old age has also
conceived a son; and this is the sixth month with her who was
called barren. 37 For with God nothing will be impossible."**

**38 And Mary said, "Behold, I am the handmaid of the Lord; let it be
to me according to your word." And the angel departed from
her.**

## ***Luke 2:1-19*** [RSV]

**1 In those days a decree went out from Caesar Augustus that all the
world should be enrolled. 2 This was the first enrollment, when
Quirinius was governor of Syria. 3 And all went to be enrolled,
each to his own city.**

**4 And Joseph also went up from Galilee, from the city of Nazareth, to
Judea, to the city of David, which is called Bethlehem, because
he was of the house and lineage of David, 5 to be enrolled with
Mary, his betrothed, who was with child.**

**6 And while they were there, the time came for her to be delivered.
7 And she gave birth to her first-born son and wrapped him in
swaddling cloths, and laid him in a manger, because there was
no place for them in the inn.**

**8 And in that region there were shepherds out in the field, keeping
watch over their flock by night.**

**9 And an angel of the Lord appeared to them, and the glory of the
Lord shone around them, and they were filled with fear. 10 And
the angel said to them, "Be not afraid; for behold, I bring you
good news of a great joy which will come to all the people; 11 for
to you is born this day in the city of David a Savior, who is
Christ the Lord. 12 And this will be a sign for you: you will find
a babe wrapped in swaddling cloths and lying in a manger."**

**13 And suddenly there was with the angel a multitude of the heavenly
host praising God and saying, 14 "Glory to God in the highest,
and on earth peace among men with whom he is pleased!"**

*Continued next page...*

15 **When the angels went away from them into heaven, the shepherds said to one another, "Let us go over to Bethlehem and see this thing that has happened, which the Lord has made known to us."**

16 **And they went with haste, and found Mary and Joseph, and the**
**babe lying in a manger. 17 And when they saw it they made**
**known the saying which had been told them concerning this**
**child; 18 and all who heard it wondered at what the shepherds**
**told them.**

19 **But Mary kept all these things, pondering them in her heart.**

## <u>Mark 15:22-39</u> [RSV]

22 **And they brought him to the place called Golgotha (which means the place of a skull).**

23 **And they offered him wine mingled with myrrh; but he did not**
**take it. 24 And they crucified him, and divided his garments**
**among them, casting lots for them, to decide what each should**
**take.**

25 **And it was the third hour, when they crucified him.**

26 **And the inscription of the charge against him read, "The King of the Jews."**

27 **And with him they crucified two robbers, one on his right and one**
**on his left. 28 *[No text]**

29 **And those who passed by derided him, wagging their heads, and**
**saying, "Aha! You who would destroy the temple and build it**
**in three days, 30 save yourself, and come down from the cross!"**

31 **So also the chief priests mocked him to one another with the**
**scribes, saying, "He saved others; he cannot save himself.**
**32 Let the Christ, the King of Israel, come down now from the**
**cross, that we may see and believe." Those who were crucified**
**with him also reviled him.**

33 **And when the sixth hour had come, there was darkness over the whole land until the ninth hour.**

**[34] And at the ninth hour Jesus cried with a loud voice, "E'lo-i, E'lo-i, la'ma sabach-tha'ni?" which means, "My God, my God, why hast thou forsaken me?"**

**[35] And some of the bystanders hearing it said, "Behold, he is calling Eli'jah." [36] And one ran and, filling a sponge full of vinegar, put it on a reed and gave it to him to drink, saying, "Wait, let us see whether Eli'jah will come to take him down."**

**[37] And Jesus uttered a loud cry, and breathed his last. [38] And the curtain of the temple was torn in two, from top to bottom.**

**[39] And when the centurion, who stood facing him, saw that he thus breathed his last, he said, "Truly this man was the Son of God!"**

## ***Matthew 28:1-10*** [RSV]

**[1] Now after the sabbath, toward the dawn of the first day of the week, Mary Magdalene and the other Mary went to see the sepulchre.**

**[2] And behold, there was a great earthquake; for an angel of the Lord descended from heaven and came and rolled back the stone,
and sat upon it. [3] His appearance was like lightning, and his
raiment white as snow. [4] And for fear of him the guards
trembled and became like dead men.**

**[5] But the angel said to the women, "Do not be afraid; for I know that
you seek Jesus who was crucified. [6] He is not here; for he has
risen, as he said. Come, see the place where he lay. [7] Then go
quickly and tell his disciples that he has risen from the dead, and behold, he is going before you to Galilee; there you will see him. Lo, I have told you."**

**[8] So they departed quickly from the tomb with fear and great joy, and ran to tell his disciples.**

**[9] And behold, Jesus met them and said, "Hail!" And they came up and took hold of his feet and worshiped him.**

**[10] Then Jesus said to them, "Do not be afraid; go and tell my brethren to go to Galilee, and there they will see me."**

## ***John 10:9-14*** [RSV]

**9 I am the door. If anyone enters by Me, he will be saved, and will go in and out and find pasture.**

**10 The thief comes only to steal and kill and destroy; I came that they may have life, and have it abundantly.**

**11 I am the good shepherd. The good shepherd lays down his life for the sheep.**

**12 He who is a hireling and not a shepherd, whose own the sheep are not, sees the wolf coming and leaves the sheep and flees; and the wolf snatches them and scatters them.**

**13 He flees because he is a hireling and cares nothing for the sheep.**

**14 I am the good shepherd; and I know My sheep, and am known by My own.**

### Here's How To Receive Jesus Into Your Life:

- Admit your need. *(I am a sinner.)*
- Be willing to turn from your sins. *(Repent.)*
- Believe that Jesus Christ died for you on the cross and rose from the grave. *(Salvation comes by faith in what Jesus did for us.)*
- Through prayer, invite Jesus Christ to control your life through the Holy Spirit. *(Receive Him as Lord and Savior.)*

**"Dear God, I know I'm a sinner, and I ask for your forgiveness. I believe Jesus Christ is Your Son. I believe He died for my sin and that you raised Him to life. I want to trust Him as my Savior and follow Him as Lord, from this day forward. Guide my life and help me to do your will. I pray this in the name of Jesus. Amen."**

# I Forgive You

***"And forgive us our debts, as we forgive our debtors."*** Matthew 6:12 [KJV]

## ***Matthew 18:21-22*** [RSV]

**21 Then Peter came up and said to him, "Lord, how often shall my brother sin against me, and I forgive him? As many as seven times?"**

**22 Jesus said to him, "I do not say to you seven times, but seventy times seven."**

## ***Matthew 5:43-48*** [RSV]

**43 You have heard that it was said, 'You shall love your neighbor and hate your enemy.'**

**44 But I say to you, Love your enemies and pray for those who**
**persecute you, 45 so that you may be sons of your Father who is**
**in heaven; for he makes his sun rise on the evil and on the good,**
**and sends rain on the just and on the unjust.**

**46 For if you love those who love you, what reward have you? Do not even the tax collectors do the same?**

**47 And if you salute only your brethren, what more are you doing than others? Do not even the Gentiles do the same?**

**48 You, therefore, must be perfect, as your heavenly Father is perfect.**

***Luke 23:33-34*** [RSV]

**33 And when they came to the place which is called
The Skull, there they crucified him, and the
criminals, one on the right and one on the left.**

**34 And Jesus said, "Father, forgive them; for they
know not what they do." And they cast lots to divide
his garments.**

***Acts 7:58-60*** [RSV]

**58 Then they cast him out of the city and stoned him; and
the witnesses laid down their garments at the feet of a
young man named Saul.**

**59 And as they were stoning Stephen, he prayed, "Lord
Jesus, receive my spirit."**

**60 And he knelt down and cried with a loud voice, "Lord, do
not hold this sin against them." And when he had said this,
he fell asleep.**

Our Father, who art in heaven, hallowed be thy name.
Let thy kingdom come and thy will be done,
on earth as it is in heaven.
Give us this day, our daily bread.
And forgive us our debts as we forgive our debtors.
Lead us not into temptation, but deliver us from evil.
For thine is the kingdom, and the power,
and the glory, forever and ever. Amen

[The Lord's Prayer, based on Matthew 6:9-13]

## ***Genesis 45:4-15*** [NKJV]

**4 And Joseph said to his brothers, "Please come near to me."
So they came near. Then he said: "I am Joseph your
brother, whom you sold into Egypt.**

**5 But now, do not therefore be grieved or angry with yourselves
because you sold me here; for God sent me before you to
preserve life. 6 For these two years the famine has been
in the land, and there are still five years in which there
will be neither plowing nor harvesting. 7 And God sent
me before you to preserve a posterity for you in the
earth, and to save your lives by a great deliverance.**

**8 So now it was not you who sent me here, but God; and He has
made me a father to Pharaoh, and lord of all his house,
and a ruler throughout all the land of Egypt.**

**9 Hurry and go up to my father, and say to him, 'Thus says
your son Joseph: "God has made me lord of all Egypt;
come down to me, do not tarry. 10 You shall dwell in the
land of Goshen, and you shall be near to me, you and
your children, your children's children, your flocks and
your herds, and all that you have. 11 There I will provide
for you, lest you and your household, and all that you
have, come to poverty; for there are still five years of
famine." ' 12 And behold, your eyes and the eyes of my
brother Benjamin see that it is my mouth that speaks to
you. 13 So you shall tell my father of all my glory in
Egypt, and of all that you have seen; and you shall hurry
and bring my father down here."**

**14 Then he fell on his brother Benjamin's neck and wept, and
Benjamin wept on his neck.**

**15 Moreover he kissed all his brothers and wept over them, and
after that his brothers talked with him.**

## *Genesis 50:15-21* [NKJV]

**15 When Joseph's brothers saw that their father was dead, they said, "Perhaps Joseph will hate us, and may actually repay us for all the evil which we did to him."**

**16 So they sent messengers to Joseph, saying, "Before your father died
he commanded, saying, 17 'Thus you shall say to Joseph: "I beg
you, please forgive the trespass of your brothers and their sin; for they did evil to you." ' Now, please, forgive the trespass of the servants of the God of your father." And Joseph wept when they spoke to him.**

**18 Then his brothers also went and fell down before his face, and they said, "Behold, we are your servants."**

**19 Joseph said to them, "Do not be afraid, for am I in the place of
God? 20 But as for you, you meant evil against me; but God
meant it for good, in order to bring it about as it is this day, to
save many people alive. 21 Now therefore, do not be afraid; I
will provide for you and your little ones." And he comforted them and spoke kindly to them.**

NOTE: Anyone who has lived for any amount of time has been hurt by someone. Sometimes it's even a person we loved deeply and cared for openly.

Some of us—if we're honest—have also had times of being disappointed with God. The following verses are included to help those struggling with spiritual disappointments … wondering where God is or was … why he didn't do as we hoped … why he allowed the opposite of our prayers to occur.

We forgive or release God—not because he needs to be forgiven—but because we need to acknowledge and confess that bitterness, anger, or doubt have flourished in the soil of our disappointment and we're choosing to let it go.

## ***Job 1:20-21*** [NKJV]

**[20] Then Job arose, tore his robe, and shaved his head; and he fell to the ground and worshiped.**

**[21] And he said: "Naked I came from my mother's womb, And naked shall I return there. The Lord gave, And the Lord has taken away; Blessed be the name of the Lord."**

## ***Job 2:9-10*** [NKJV]

**[9] Then his wife said to him, "Do you still hold fast to your integrity? Curse God and die!"**

**[10] But he said to her, "You speak as one of the foolish women speaks. Shall we indeed accept good from God, and shall we not accept adversity?" In all this Job did not sin with his lips.**

## ***Job 19:23-27*** [KJV]

**[23] Oh, that my words were written! Oh, that they were**
**inscribed in a book! [24] That they were engraved on a rock with**
**an iron pen and lead, forever!**

**[25] For I know that my Redeemer lives, And He shall stand at**
**last on the earth; [26] And after my skin is destroyed, this I know,**
**that in my flesh I shall see God,**

**[27] Whom I shall see for myself, And my eyes shall behold, and not another. How my heart yearns within me!**

## ***Isaiah 55:8-9*** [MSG]

**[8] "I don't think the way you think. The way you work isn't the way I work." God's Decree.**

**[9] "For as the sky soars high above earth, so the way I work surpasses the way you work, and the way I think is beyond the way you think...."**

## ***Isaiah 45:9-11*** [NIV]

**9 "Woe to those who quarrel with their Maker, those who are nothing but potsherds among the potsherds on the ground. Does the clay say to the potter, 'What are you making?' Does your work say, 'The potter has no hands?'**

**10 Woe to the one who says to a father, 'What have you begotten?' or to a mother, 'What have you brought to birth?'**

**11 "This is what the LORD says—the Holy One of Israel, and its Maker: Concerning things to come, do you question me about my children, or give me orders about the work of my hands?"**

## ***1 Peter 5:6-11*** [RSV]

**6 Humble yourselves therefore under the mighty hand of God, that in due time he may exalt you.**

**7 Cast all your anxieties on him, for he cares about you.**

**8 Be sober, be watchful. Your adversary the devil prowls around like a roaring lion, seeking some one to devour.**

**9 Resist him, firm in your faith, knowing that the same experience of suffering is required of your brotherhood throughout the world.**

**10 And after you have suffered a little while, the God of all grace, who has called you to his eternal glory in Christ, will himself restore, establish, and strengthen you.**

**11 To him be the dominion for ever and ever. Amen.**

## ***Psalm 22:1-11*** [NIV]

**1 My God, my God, why have you forsaken me? Why are you so far from saving me, so far from my cries of anguish?**

**2 My God, I cry out by day, but you do not answer, by night, but I find no rest.**

**3 Yet you are enthroned as the Holy One; you are the one Israel**
**praises. 4 In you our ancestors put their trust; they**
**trusted and you delivered them. 5 To you they cried out**
**and were saved; in you they trusted and were not put to shame.**

**6 But I am a worm and not a man, scorned by everyone, despised**
**by the people. 7 All who see me mock me; they hurl**
**insults, shaking their heads.**

**8 "He trusts in the LORD," they say, "let the LORD rescue him. Let him deliver him, since he delights in him."**

**9 Yet you brought me out of the womb; you made me trust in**
**you, even at my mother's breast. 10 From birth I was cast**
**on you; from my mother's womb you have been my God.**

**11 Do not be far from me, for trouble is near and there is no one to help.**

# How Great Thou Art

Oh Lord my God! When I in awesome wonder,
consider all the worlds Thy hands have made.
I see the stars, I hear the rolling thunder,
Thy power throughout the universe displayed.

When through the woods and forest glades I wander,
and hear the birds sing sweetly in the trees.
When I look down from lofty mountain grandeur,
and hear the brook and feel the gentle breeze.

And when I think that God, His Son not sparing,
sent Him to die, I scarce can take it in;
that on the cross, my burden gladly bearing,
He bled and died to take away my sin.

When Christ shall come with shout of acclamation,
and take me home, what joy shall fill my heart!
Then I shall bow in humble adoration,
and there proclaim, my God, how great Thou art.

***Refrain:***

Then sings my soul, my Savior God to Thee;
how great Thou art, how great Thou art!
Then sings my soul, My Savior God to Thee;
how great Thou art, how great Thou art!

Words and music by
Carl G. Boberg & R.J. Hughes

# Section Two
## *Stories*

This section includes the voices of those who once stood where you stand now.

**Some of these stories were collected for an anthropology research** project in 2000. For that project, I interviewed 18 individuals who had received a terminal diagnosis and/or someone who cared for a terminal patient during their last days. The analysis of those interviews completed a thesis requirement for San Jose State, revealed new ways to meet the non-medical needs of hospice patients, and accidentally formed the foundation for a not-for-profit business called *Legacies* (dedicated to preserving the significant memories of ordinary people).

Participants' stories were tape-recorded, transcribed, and organized for ease of reading. They told their stories, in the first person—they were not stories about them. Since the participants stated they hoped their experience would help others, I included their stories in the appendix of the thesis and have reprinted applicable portions for you to read here (with written permission). At the end of this section, you'll find a list of the questions I used to initiate the therapeutic reminiscing examined in the study.

The study—as well as personal experiences with terminal patients—has convinced me:

- Dying people benefit from being heard (social reminiscing)
- Dying people benefit from assurances they'll be remembered

The names from the San Jose State Research have been changed to protect the privacy of participants. Since their stories surround significant memories and the objects that marked those memories, I've included some pictures of their treasures. Enclosed transcripts are reprinted with permission from *Legacies: How People Transform Memories Into Memorials*.

**For the Second Edition**, I included stories from friends and family. These individuals also signed consent forms; however, these narrators asked me to include their names.

**Daily Survival Kit for Serious Illness**
By Thomas L. McDermitt
A long-time cancer patient and skeptic

- Today I am going to try to live through this day only, and not dwell on or attempt to solve all my problems at once; just focus on the piece that is today. I can do something for several hours that would be difficult to even think about continuing for several months.

- Just for today, I am willing to accept the possibility that there is a purpose to this suffering; that it can be a source of meaning and growth for myself and others, though I may not always recognize the ways. And it seems possible that this suffering will not be in vain, because of what may be some of kind existence beyond.

- Today I may feel the need to complain a great deal; I may have little tolerance; I may cry; I may scream. That does not mean that I am less courageous or strong. All are ways of expressing anger over this mess, of rightly mourning my losses. Endurance itself is courage.

- Surviving this is all so difficult. At times it seems impossible—that I have had enough. Down the line I will know if and when I have had enough, when I cannot push the limits any further. I will have the right to choose to stop, without feeling that I am "giving up." But today I think I can deal with this illness. Sorrow runs very deep, but I think I can rise again.

- Just for today, perhaps I can take heart that we are all connected. And I may still have some things left to contribute to the family of man; some light to add to the light. Even now my endurance (however imperfect) is a gift, an inspiration for others in their struggles.

- It seems reasonable that there is a season for everything, and a time for every purpose. Pain, weakness and exhaustion may distort my sense and spirit. Today, however, I can at least find some hope in nature's way, if not in some master plan. The chances are fairly good, and it seems worthwhile to hope that I will have some cycle of wellness yet.

**NOTE from the compiler.** Thomas McDermitt wrote this Daily Survival Kit in 1989 for those battling acute or chronic illnesses. There are ten bullet points in his essay but I only included the ones that might benefit a hospice patient or caregiver.

They are unedited or adapted; they are typed exactly as he wrote them.

For the entire essay, do an online search for "Daily Survival Kit" by Thomas McDermitt. It will come up on many websites.

> *The hardest thing for me to talk about, the hardest thing for me to go through, was to watch her suffer. It's the hardest thing I've ever done in my life.*

### *Tony*

**Caregiver for his wife, Nan**
**Nan was the inspiration for this book**

I knew when we got married she wasn't going to live a long time, that she would die young. I had a premonition we weren't going to grow old together and she used to say the same thing to me. That was when she was healthy and full of energy, before she was diagnosed. So, when it happened, I wasn't surprised. It's a blow, but inside you're thinking, *well, unfortunately, I was right.*

I can't remember how it started. I think she had a soreness in her arm or felt a lump and went in to have it checked—that's when she found out she had cancer. When she was first diagnosed, I knew it could be terminal, but I had no idea how long it would last. She lived another 12 ½ years after being diagnosed.

The first seven or eight years weren't too bad. Lots of going in and out of the hospital, lots of doctor care and appointments. Some people caring, some people not so much. She had one season when she almost went five years. She was praying for that fifth year to get by because she wanted to say she was cured. And … just as she was getting close to the fifth year, it popped up again and we had to go back and do the whole thing all over again.

It was so hard to see her go through it, go through the pain. The hardest thing for me to tell you about, the hardest thing for me to go through, was to watch her suffer. It's the hardest thing I've ever done in my life.

Another hard thing was watching her lose so many things. Losing life. Losing the ability to drive a car, losing the ability to do the books or pay the bills, losing the ability to have any stamina to do any little thing. She used to love to cook, and then she didn't have the strength to cook. We always ate the evening meal together. She lost that—couldn't sit at the table and eat dinner. Through a series of steps, she lost her grasp on life. I remember her crying when she lost the ability to do something else, every loss—no matter how little—was very traumatic.

Up till the month before she died, I did all of the caregiving. I kept our children out of it as much as I could because I didn't want them to have bad memories of their mother. I didn't want them to have to watch her go through this. But, as the time ended, I felt that they needed to know what was going on. It was time.

I asked each of them to help take care of her. I made a schedule and they all agreed to come and help take care of their mom so I could get away for a few days. One of the boys was here for 12 hours and couldn't spend the night like he was supposed to. He called his brother and said, 'I can't do this.' My oldest son came and stayed the night for him.

She wanted to die in our bed but I couldn't make that happen; in the end, we had to bring in a hospital bed. She did get to die at home—that's what she wanted.

I learned a lot from her and with her. In a way, we grew up together. We had a lot of fun—she was a great companion. It's been three years and I still miss her today.

### *Debbie*

**Caregiver for her father**

> *His whole life, he always thought it would be really cool if he could drop dead on the dance floor or the tennis courts or something. That was his definition of a good death—good health, having fun and drop dead.*

My dad told us something was *going on* but was very close-mouthed about the whole thing. He was very vague, very left-handed when it came to explaining. I was trying to get information and he didn't seem to want to or wasn't able to give it. I asked him questions and I'd get a lot of shoulder shrugging and toe digging.

Sometime later, he asked me to go to the doctor with him. So, I said, "OK" and went with my questions. The nurse told me where to get some booklets from the library so I could read about non-Hodgkins Lymphoma.

I picked up the pamphlets, came home, and read them. It said there are two distinct groups of people when it comes to this diagnosis: Some want to know everything and be totally involved in every decision; the others don't want to know any more than they have to. The booklet said: However your loved one views their illness, the important thing is to respect how they're viewing it. If they don't want to know more, you can offer, "Would you like to read this?" But if they say, "No", throw it away.

That sounded like good advice. My dad was the kind that said, "I don't want to know anything. I don't want to talk about it."

He took the treatments when his doctor told him to. He had some surgery and some chemotherapy. Over the last couple of years, he had many, many rounds of the kind of chemo you take for his disease. He took it orally, at home.

The disease progressed in steps. There were five years that were pretty good; he had some treatments but was doing okay. Then he dropped down to where the treatments were more regular.

Eventually—I don't know the date and I don't really remember what prompted it—but I ended up on the phone with his doctor.

She told me, "Well, we're at a point where it's time to make some decisions."

I said, "What kind of decisions?"

"It may come to the point where he no longer wants treatment because the treatment is worse than the disease and when you get to that point, you may want to make some other choices. I'd like you to come in with him and we'll talk about some options."

That's when I knew he wasn't going to beat it. Of course, I burst into tears and called my boyfriend. Got him on the phone, he's crying. I'm sitting at work, we're all crying. I'm saying, "This is it. This is it."

We all went to the next doctor's visit because the doctor said to bring anyone who would be involved in caring for him. I went and so did my boyfriend and my sister. The doctor said to all of us, "Well, if he goes hospice, we'll need someone to be the primary caregiver."

You could've heard all the heads turn, I mean you could have heard it, they all turned and looked at me. So I said, "I guess it's me."

Leaving that day, my dad knew, he understood what we were talking about. On the way home, he broke down and cried. I felt so bad .... but other than that time—I mean he was upset that day but then it was right back to where he was. He never really talked about the big deep meaning of life. He just pulled himself together and he looked at me and said, "You're going to love that car."

I told him, "Yea, I will."

No one came to visit him once he became homebound. No one. Just us. I asked him while he was still fairly talkative if he wanted me to call his sister.

"Should I call your sister? Would you like her to come over?"

He was, "No, no. Don't call her."

I asked him if I should call anybody. He kept saying, "No." And the message I got, I don't really know if he said it or I inferred it, but the message I heard was, 'I don't want anybody to see me like this.' That's the message I heard.

His whole life, he always thought it would be really cool if he could drop dead on the dance floor or the tennis courts. I used to tell him, "You want to upset everyone around you?" But he felt like that was the way to go. That's his definition of a good death: good health, having fun, and drop dead. I think that's why he chose hospice, he wasn't interested in life-saving procedures, he didn't want to be hooked up and barely alive. He didn't think it was being alive if machines were doing the work.

I've made a conscious effort to not remember most of the stuff that happened during the last months. It's not how you want to remember a person. I can remember certain things quite clearly because you could just never forget them.

One time … Two weeks before he died, he was in terrible shape, but he insisted that he go fishing. I thought, *Oh God, this is a man who is incontinent, can barely get around, weak, thin, sick, can't eat, a mess—and he wants to go fishing!* He wanted to go out on a party boat. Out on the ocean. He wanted to hold a fishing pole in his hands one more time.

My boyfriend said he'd take him out on one of those little boats that go out of Half Moon Bay. It was a disaster from the start. It was a miserable, miserable trip. He could barely hold the rod, he couldn't really fish. He laid down, he was in the bathroom ... he didn't have a very good time. But he did it. I think that's when he decided that it was over. 'If I can't go fishing anymore, what's the point?'

One day the hospice nurse said she could tell from his breathing that it wouldn't be long—when the breathing changes, they know it's close. I called my son and told him to leave school and come. He came down. We were all there around his hospital bed. This was probably the nice part. My son played his guitar. We all talked to him; he could hear us because he would nod, but he didn't talk. He knew we were there. It was like, when my son got there, he knew it was OK—I think he might have been waiting to see my son once more. So that was amazing.

He had arranged to be cremated by the Neptune Society. He wanted it that way, all arranged so that I didn't have to do anything. They came and picked him up and cremated him. Then we went to visit them and filled out all the paperwork, lots and lots of paperwork.

Then she said, "These are your choices for the ashes."

I was stumped, I didn't know I would have choices. She was really nice and very sensitive. I don't remember all the choices, but I do know that he was entitled to a military burial because he had served in the military. I didn't think the military was that important to him. They did give me the flag just because he was in the service (they mailed it to me).

She told me that there were boats that go all over and do the sea scattering. The other one is a selection of party fishing boats that go out of Half Moon Bay. I said, "Let me see the names." I saw the name of the boat he always went fishing on, Captain Jack's. I told her, "I want that boat."

They arranged everything. We went out in the afternoon, it was a beautiful, calm day. We went out on the fishing boat and cruised around; they have rules about putting ashes out to sea, you have to be out a certain distance from the shore.

I had my boyfriend do it, I couldn't do it. I think my son scattered the last of them. Someone might have said something, but I couldn't tell you what. Then we cruised around some more. We were the only ones on the boat. The crew remembered him. *Crotchety old guy with European-American hair.*

I do feel pretty good in that I did all that I could do. I know some people have to deal with, "I should have done this or that," or, "I should have done more" but I don't really have that feeling. I feel like I did OK. I have some sad things to look back on but I feel good about others. I try not to focus on the hard times.

### *Diana*
**Caregiver for her husband**

The last year we had together was a precious time … We did a lot of laughing. I tried to do things that we used to do. Then there were things that we *needed* to do. I'm so thankful for that year. It was a precious time that we had. He just wanted me with him all the time.

I'd wash his feet. I'd put this special cream on them and massage them. His feet needed to be massaged because he would swell in the ankles, so I'd try to keep the swelling down by massaging them. Every week, we had stuff we had to do, doctor's appointments. We were together all the time and it was good.

There were times when he said things he needed to say. Me too. He said, "I'm sorry for this and that." And I said, "I'm sorry for this and that." Just clean the deck. Leave nothing unsaid. That's the beauty of being able to let it go.

He was able to tell me what to do about things that would need to get done when he was gone. He tried to get me ready, prepare me. He knew it was getting near the end. We both knew.

*After he raised his hand and looked to the door, he just started to breath really slow. And then ... he was gone. We said, "Bye, Tom. Bye. See you in heaven."*

## ***Jean***

**Caregiver for her son, Tom**

Tom was very outgoing. He was the one who came in singing, slamming the door—you knew when he was home. And Abe, our youngest son, was always quiet. That was the difference between the two.

During Tom's first year in college, he found a lump on his back. It hurt so the doctor took it out. It took a while for the HMO to Ok the tests to find out what it was. It was a Schwannoma, it's a Schwann cell which is a nerve cell that went awry somehow. The diagnosis was that it was benign. But they didn't realize that underneath the benign one was a malignant one. So, we thought everything was fine.

Then, it started to come up again. They didn't know if it was a hematoma that had occurred in the area of the first operation or if it was indeed another tumor. And because of different things, it wasn't caught in time.

Meanwhile, he went on a mission trip to Spain. I think he just figured if God was going to heal him, he would heal him. If He didn't want to, he wouldn't. That was about it. That's what he said, but who knows what he felt inside. You know what I mean? I never saw him get angry, angry with the doctors or angry with God.

I do remember one time when we were driving to the doctor's office, early in the whole situation, and he said, "Why me? Why not a drug addict on the streets of San Francisco? Why is it me?"

I didn't have an answer. But, he made peace with the Lord over those things. It WAS him, and that's the way it was. He dealt with that.

One memory that I have that's precious to me .... He'd been in UCSF for 57 days for a lung operation, to try and get rid of cancerous spots on his lungs. Just as we were getting ready to leave the hospital, I noticed he had another lump on his back. I didn't want to tell him, but I had to. We had to get it checked.

We had an MRI on it and we found out it was a tumor that was pressing on his spine. They were very concerned about that and we had to go directly to the hospital and get radiation THAT day. And then they said, if there's any weakness in his legs, you need to bring him right back in. They said they wouldn't normally let him go home but because I was going to be with him, they let him go home.

We were on our way home. He said, "Well, I guess we better get a bunch of people together to pray tonight."

So he starts organizing it all. He said, "Dad, why don't we drop you off and you call everyone to come pray. Mom, let's go over and get a Nintendo set, I think it's time for me to have it."

So I took him over to Toys R Us, and we went in ... I was afraid he was going to fall, he was that weak. We went in and he chose the one he wanted. I stood in line and he went out. I really didn't want him to go out to the car by himself, but I felt that was something he needed to do. So he went out by himself and I stood in line and got it.

Then, we're coming back over the hill, over Serra Monte Hill. You come over a short part of it and then you drop down to this beautiful vista of the Pacific Ocean. He had this Nintendo Set on his lap ... Steven Curtis Chapman or somebody is singing "For Him" from the car stereo. We're singing this song with him and coming into this view.

I thought to myself, *I'm never going to forget this.* There was no self-pity, there was no downer. We're worshipping the Lord, he has this thing on his lap, and we're going home to pray with anyone who will come. It was precious, precious ....

Let me tell you about the night he died … to me that's important.

Through the day—it was Easter Sunday—through the day, he was going in and out of consciousness. He said some things that we talked about before. "I can't take a drink because I'm getting married today." Another time, he said, "Call all my friends and have them come over because I want to show them who I really am."

So, we called all his friends, and they came. This was in the afternoon. He didn't go into the coma until about seven that night, maybe eight.

When he went into a coma, he stopped breathing briefly but my husband revived him. We felt it was timc to call Molly, thc hospice nurse.

When she got there, she said, "Why don't you put him in the recliner that you have in his room. We'll make him as comfortable as we can because we don't really know how long he'll be in this situation. But, probably, he can hear everything you say."

So we put him in the recliner. His friends began to come. They filled the back room. There were two young people with guitars and they were singing Christian songs. They were praying and talking to him. It was so awesome. It felt good. It felt like the presence of the Lord was there but it didn't feel like oooooh—spooky. It just felt comfortable.

We didn't know how soon it was going to be at first. It wasn't like people were saying 'goodbye' yet. But then his breathing was getting slower. I knew that his death was near. So his dad went in and said something to him. I went in at one point and talked to him. Abe was right by him, holding his hand and talking to him. His friends were there and they were talking and singing. It was just going on like that.

Then, someone called to me and said, "Come on back, come back here because he raised his hand up and looked toward the door."

He hadn't done anything up till then. After that, he just started to breathe really slow. And then he was gone. People were calling, "Bye, Tom. See you in heaven."

We all went out into the living room, formed a huge circle, and sang praise songs.

Finally, we called the mortuary and told them to come. They were totally blown away. They said, "We walk in homes and we're usually spat at or hit or yelled at or sworn at—this is unbelievable. Are you sure someone's dead in here?" That was about 4 in the morning.

Those months with him at home were really precious. But not any more than any other time with him. I enjoyed him all the time. Those were hard times because there was a lot of hard stuff. I remember one morning, going to the hospital for him to have that big operation on both his lungs. We just sat in the room and cried. What was there to do? We just cried and prayed.

You don't see his things around the house. We cleaned out his room. Tom died at Easter and Abe was coming home for the summer. He said, "I can't sleep in that room."

So we took everything out, repainted, and put different stuff back in—we made it Abe's room. It wasn't that we wanted to get rid of Tom's things, to keep the things in there as they were would not be good. It wouldn't be fair to Abe. So we redid it. Completely changed it. And then, after Abe graduated and moved out, I decided that I needed MY place. So now, I've turned it into my prayer closet.

***Dan***

**WWII veteran, Battle of the Bulge, D-1 Day**
**Firefighter shot in the line of duty**

My friend and I enlisted in the army before the war broke out. We were based in Tennessee together but when we got sent overseas, we got split up.

I was in the group that was set to land in Normandy on D-1, not D-Day, but D-1. I remember it very vividly. On D-day, we left England and went across the English Channel. The next day, eleven o'clock at night, on D-1, we went in.

Then you're scared. The battleships were shooting over us—the Missouri—they were shooting the big guns over our heads. It was chaos.

We went down the big ship on rope ladders and got into the landing craft. We went as far as they could take us and then waded the rest of the way in … the water was halfway up to our knees.

Our commander told us, "Just dig a hole on the beach and we'll get organized in the morning."

There were already lots of foxholes there from the night before but if you couldn't find one, you had to dig your own.

When I woke up the next morning … they had a wire-fenced area—about 10 X 10 feet. They'd captured a couple of Germans on the beach and they were in this temporary prison. One guy tried to get out and they shot him. So he was just there, hanging on the wires. That's the first thing I saw when I woke up in the morning—there's a dead guy laying in the wires.

So in the morning, we got organized and they told us what our mission would be. The General was there and he told us we were supposed to climb to the top of a hill in Normandy … Then he said, "Now, I'm going to tell you, half of you ain't coming back."

You're just kids, you know? You're 21 and they're telling you, "Half of you ain't gonna make it." He said it like it was. He wanted us ready. His message was clear, 'Say your prayers because this could be it.'

My unit was in Normandy for the first eleven days … later, I was in the Battle of the Bulge on the ambulance crew. I think back to all we went through in the war—all the harrowing escapes—maybe I should say close calls. During the day, we spent the whole day in our trench with planes coming over us. The ground just shook, we could see the bombs coming down. While the bombing was going on, we had to be in our holes.

You couldn't think that you were going to be the one who didn't make it. You had to think, "We've got a job and we're going to do it."

…. I made it home without injury.

When I got out and home, I joined the Milwaukee Fire Department. It was 1948 (my father had been the chief and I always wanted to follow in his footsteps). I loved the excitement and the camaraderie. I was one of those firefighters you see with icicles hanging off their helmets. Lots of close calls for me and the men I worked with ….

I think the biggest turning point in my life came when I was shot, in the fire department. We weren't even supposed to be in that area. My brother-in-law was at a fire about two blocks away and all the companies responded there. Then the next alarm came in and we responded and had to fill in for them.

As we're going down the street, we could see the sky was red already. At that time, we didn't have to wear rubber coats or anything, just jackets. But I had a brand new rubber coat that I'd just bought, two days earlier. I said, "I better put this on, it looks like a good worker." So I put it on.

We got to the fire and the front end of the building, a two-story building, was going wide open. So the chief told me to take my company and come from the alley. He thought maybe we could get into the building that way.

So we broke the back door down and got in there. We didn't know at first, but there was a fellow living in that warehouse. I don't know how he could live in there, but he was. He was asleep in a car when we entered.

So we came in through the alley and we're crawling on the floor beneath the smoke to see what we could see. I was the officer so I went first with a flashlight and was trying to see. Eventually, I came to this truck, or parked vehicle in there.

I felt my way around it and when I got to the window, the guy living in there reached out the window and shot his gun at the light. He was about three feet away from me. He hit me right in the chest. It knocked me down, flatter than a pancake.

Two guys behind me said, "What was that?"

I said, "I'm shot."

So they grabbed me by the collar and dragged me out. I was laying on the ground but I was conscious.

I was shocked. The police were at the alarm anyway, so they called for an ambulance. Our ambulance was at the other fire. The police said, "Well, we got an ambulance right here."

So they threw me in the ambulance and carted me out to the county hospital. I spent the next three months there—91 days.

The head doctor that took care of me, said, "I've lost a lot easier ones than you."

The bullet went right into the chest and then tore up the stomach, the liver, the lungs, and the bowels—it lodged in the back of them. They took out the bullet, removed it from the back. It shattered when it hit my breastbone. Pieces of it went everywhere.

They had to remove part of my stomach and part of the liver that was damaged. The bowels, I had a colostomy for the whole time I was in the hospital.

They wanted me to go home and rest awhile and come back to undo the colostomy later, but I said, "No, I come here in one piece and I want to go home in one piece. I want this taken care of before I go home."

I figured that I was going to make it, but it was still a major turning point for me. I started taking life more seriously. I realized that life could be short, real short. I just thought about things differently....

*Dan recovered from the damage but because of it, battled infections the rest of his life. Eventually, it took a toll on his heart and he died. He was a kind man with the best smile. Loved by everyone who knew him.*

## *Marcy*
**Caregiver for her mother**

> *I always say, "When you get a chance, tell people you love 'em."*

My mother was 47 when she was first diagnosed with ovarian cancer. I was married. I had two children and the third one was on the way.

As the disease progressed, they requested family members to come and help. In those days, they didn't have anything like hospice. So the last six months, I helped. I spent three months, living right there. I had a baby. I mean, I was changing my baby's diaper, I laid her on the bed and changed her diaper, and then changed my mom's diaper. My other two were running around; there were some kids in the neighborhood that they'd play with. I just had to do what I could to help my mom.

She was only 49 when she died. She died alone. She was in her home, but she was alone. She didn't talk about the fact that she was dying. She wouldn't talk about it. It was so sad, you would go into the room and you would talk about the weather, talk about anything but her situation. We had so much unresolved stuff and I wanted so much to .... but I didn't have it in me to force it on her at the time. Death was definitely a subject that she wanted to avoid.

One day when I was leaving, there was a neighbor in with her, talking to her. I wanted the neighbor to leave so I could talk to my mother before I left, I wanted to have a proper goodbye with my mom. The neighbor started to leave and my mom said, "Oh no, no, no. I want you to stay." She didn't want to talk to me alone. She didn't want to talk to me on that level of saying goodbye.

I still sit back and think, "I should have said, 'Sorry, ma'am, could you leave?" That's what I should have said, but I didn't. I didn't have the tools at the time that I have now. So we never talked about her dying; two days later, she died. She died without anything being resolved.

So years later, when my grandfather was dying, I thought, *That's never going to happen again.* We only lived about two hours away so we'd visit him on the weekends.

One time I went to see him, and I hadn't seen him in a week and a half, and he had really failed badly. So I walked back there and I started to cry. And I said, "Oh, you look so bad. I'm so sad that you don't look good and I don't want to lose you. I love you."

My daughter is like, "Mom don't talk like that."

I said, "This is the way I feel and I want to share it with him. He doesn't look good. I'm not going to say that he does. I'm not going to talk about the weather."

I cried. He cried. I can still see my mascara all over the sheets and all over his pajamas.

He broke down and cried. He hugged me. I said, "I don't want to lose you. I appreciate everything you've done for me. If it wouldn't have been for you, I wouldn't have had a father."

He patted me on my back. I hugged him. I hurt so bad because I could never do that with my mom. I was determined to be real with him. Everybody looked at me like, *I can't believe she's in there crying all over him.* I didn't care what they thought.

Do you know that after he died, everything was OK? I didn't have any unfinished business. That's something I learned.

I tell people when you get a chance, tell people you love 'em. My experience with my mother where we couldn't talk about it, leaves you haunted. If I could go back ... God, if I could go back. I could have made her life so much ... I could have given her so much joy if I had found the courage to tell her how much she meant to me. But I didn't.

So, my lifelong goal is to tell everyone, "If you have a chance, tell people you care about that you love them. Tell them goodbye."

*There's people that have their children until they're fifty, sixty, seventy years old and they sometimes don't have what Jamie and I had in 28 years. They don't have that because they don't have to. They figure, "Oh well, we've got tomorrow." We didn't have tomorrow, we had to do today. We had to get everything that we could do, done today. And that's what we did. It was a real gift.*

## *Shirley*

**Caregiver for her 28-year-old son**

The first close person I lost to death was my son. I got into gardening after he died … I think it helped a lot with my mental state.

It began with some numbness in his little finger and headaches. He was 27 when it started. He went to the doctor and the doctor diagnosed him as being depressed.

One day he came home from work and said, "Mom, I'm really sick."

He looked like a stroke patient. His mouth was drooped on one side, he was dragging a leg, and his arm was kind of bent up.

I called the doctor and he said, "Bring him down."

They did a brain scan and it showed there was something there that shouldn't be. The doctor came in and apologized to us. He said, "I'm so sorry, Jamie, there really is something wrong." They put him in the hospital.

Then they sent us up to San Francisco for a brain biopsy. When we got there, the surgeon didn't want to do the biopsy. He said if they did the biopsy, Jamie might be in worse shape than he already was.

So we made a couple of trips between doctors, and the third time we went up to San Francisco, Jamie said, "I want to know what's wrong."

So they did the biopsy on June 31st. They bored into his brain in a couple of places and took pieces of it for biopsies. The cancer he had was very, very fast-growing. And very invasive. The cells, from what I understand, split and multiplied every six to ten days. It's a bad one. There's no cure for it.

The doctor called me in and told me it was brain cancer and he wouldn't make it. He said, "You're going to have a lot of people that are going to give you a lot of hype. But, I'm telling you right now, he's not going to make it."

They did this procedure in Palo Alto. After the biopsy, I stayed until late but had to get home to get ready to bring him home. I don't really remember driving home. I was crying so hard, I don't know how I got home—but I did.

I woke up about three o'clock in the morning and called up there. They said he'd had a massive seizure but he's "Ok." So I brought him home the next day.

Jamie told me, "Mom, I didn't know anybody, but I knew Jesus."

To this day, I wonder if God didn't let him live to give us more time. We only had seven months with him after that biopsy.

He was part of a research group at the University of San Francisco. He was Number 48. He took a lot of new drugs and they ran a lot of MRI's to see if it helped. He did the chemo and radiation too. He knew he wouldn't live. But he was hoping this research would help somebody else. Jamie knew from the beginning he was going to die. We just didn't know when.

We did have a lot of good times .... We went to the beach—when he got to where he couldn't walk anymore, I took him in a wheelchair. We did a lot of things together. We had a lot of fun. At first, he was able to walk with a cane. Then with a four-pronged cane. Each day, he progressively got worse and worse and worse until he was in a wheelchair. And then, toward the end, he couldn't even sit in a wheelchair without being tied in.

He could say a few words. The last time that I took him up to see his daughter, we were coming home and I said, "Would you like to have a milkshake?"

He said, "Yeah."

So we drove in ... now he looked outside the window of the car and there were a lot of poppies growing out there ... and he said just as clear as he could, "Poppies." And it was just like ... every little thing he said was music to my ears. It was such a gift. He was able, up until the time that he died, to say, "I love you." He'd say, "I love you." That was his whole sentence.

I don't know if you've ever said the little prayer of "Now I lay me down to sleep..." Well, he would say that prayer every night. When it got to where he couldn't say it anymore, then I would help him with it. And when he couldn't say it at all, I'd ask him, "Do you want me to say it for you." He'd nod "yes" that he wanted me to say it for him. So I'd say it for him every night.

We had so much time. When I think back, there are people that have their children until they're fifty, sixty, seventy years old, and the mother's still alive. They sometimes don't have what Jamie and I had in 28 years. They don't have that because they don't have to. They figure, "Oh well, we've got tomorrow, we've got tomorrow, we've got tomorrow." We didn't have tomorrow. We had to do today. We had to get everything that we could do, done today. And that's what we did. It was a real gift. It was a hard time but it was a gift of time.

Jamie wasn't in any pain. He was on no pain medication. That was such a blessing.

When Jamie died, we had an experience … well, I just don't think is normal. The night before he died, I'd say, maybe about 5 o'clock in the morning or so, I was sitting by his bed and I heard the angels singing in my ears. I looked up and ... whether it was an angel or whether it was my mother, I don't know ... but it looked just like my mother. And she had her arms held out like this for him. [Shows me that she's holding out her arms as if to say, "Come with me."] I could hear the singing.

A peace came over me. I went upstairs and got my husband and said, "You're not going to believe what happened." I told him the story.

That evening, my friend said, "You've got to lay down and rest because you'll be up tonight."

He was in a coma for the last four days, but they told me that sometimes people can still hear when they're in a coma. So I had been reading to him and talking to him. So when she came, she said, "I'll read, you go get some sleep."

When she left at 4:30, I went in to see him. I saw Jamie move, just his arm. It was the first movement he'd made since he went into the coma. I said, "Larry, something's happening. I think he's dying right now."

So my husband put, "Peace in the Valley" by Tennessee Ernie Ford on the stereo and we just held him. He took a couple of breaths and was gone.

Then I called everyone and told them if they wanted to come and see him, to come. He was going to be cremated so if they didn't come then, they wouldn't get to see him.

There were so many things that happened. Spiritual things and things that you can't really explain. Not only to me, but to other people too.

I have so many happy memories. There's not a day goes by that I don't miss him. I lost ... the thing that I lost outside of losing my son ... is I lost my joy. There was a joy that died with Jamie that I've never gotten back. I'm happy. But there is a certain little point of my joy that went with Jamie and I don't think I'll ever have it again. But, talking about him doesn't seem to hurt me. It doesn't make me miss him more or make me miss him less. It's just ... it's nice for people to know who he was.

### *Janniece*

**Breast cancer**

**Died at the age of 52 in August 2003**

.... It's like, all of a sudden you have to think about your mortality when you don't want to. It's the last thing you want to think about. All of us. Nobody wants to think about dying. We all think we're going to live forever. Something's going to happen, you know, I won't die. The world can't spin around without ME. Well, we cancer patients are fully aware that it could happen. I just don't see me going real quick.

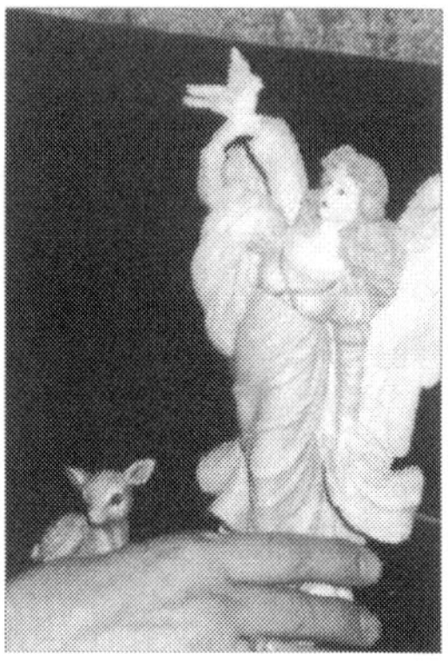

.... I started collecting angels because my best friend was collecting them. This was before '96. Then I thought, "This is cool." Now a lot of people collect them. But when you're going through crap like I'm going through, it's very comforting.

***NOTES*** from the compiler of this book, I had the honor of being one of her caregivers...

To Janniece, the angels in her collection weren't just pretty objects but tangible symbols that somebody cared and she was not alone. This was her favorite angel because it was from her sister and it looked like her when she had hair.

Janniece got into a trial test program in San Francisco in the last six months of her life. I was her designated driver. We'd drive up every three weeks, find a parking spot, and go up to the infusion floor in the Susan B Anthony Hospital for treatment. In the beginning, we'd do some minor shopping close by before her treatment. Toward the end, we'd make a bed for her in the back seat of my car before we left her home. She'd crawl into her little cave of quilts ... sometimes talking to me on the way up but often just dozing fitfully. I remember the tears the day they told her she could no longer participate in the trial because her health was failing too much. All I heard on the ride home was quiet sobs.

She started seeing a local oncologist for weekly blood work. Again, I was her designated driver. On the last visit, she wanted me in the room with her ... I suspect she knew it wasn't going to go well. The doctor told her as calmly, quietly, and slowly as he could ... that he'd ordered a wheelchair to take her over to the hospital, she needed to be admitted.

She was beyond tears at that point, she was angry. She did not want to die and did not want anyone to even hint she wouldn't make it. But they wheeled her over to the hospital. I moved the car to another parking lot and came in to find her room.

For four days, she fought death. They said if no one would sit with her, she'd have to be restrained because she was determined to leave the hospital. Three of us took shifts sitting with her 24 hours a day so she wouldn't need to be strapped down.

It was my turn at her bedside the day she died. She could no longer talk or open her eyes. And then suddenly, she took a deep breath of air. Her eyes flew open and she looked at me. Her eyes closed and she sighed and sighed and sighed until there was no more breath to sigh. Her battle with breast cancer was over.

She was always a feisty, fun lady. Tiny and pretty with long blonde hair. I'm glad I was the friend who didn't work full-time, glad I got to spend time with her as she battled, glad I was with her when she left. I consider it the last gift she gave me.

***Carl***

**A caregiver for his mother**
**and shared about several of his terminal diagnoses**
**He died in June of 2004**

> *People shouldn't have to wait until they're dead to have nice things said about them.*

Every life has a story to tell—some people are just more capable of presenting it ... I don't have any big stories to tell. I've never done anything with any significance. I'll never write a book—I don't have the ability or the intelligence or the education. You have to be trained to do something like that right….

I remember very significant things in my life because I've gone over them so many times. I remember the past more than I do the present. I can do something today and I don't even remember it tomorrow. But I can go back to when I was six years old and in the Shriner's hospital—seventy years ago. I can still see that old hospital there, where I was, how sunny it was, how the sun used to come through the windows….

At the age of 76, I shouldn't have lived this long, but I'm here for some reason. I asked my mother one time, "Mama, why am I still at home with you?"

She said, "God gave you to me so that you could take care of me."

My mother was a good woman, a sweet woman, a kind woman. Never had anything bad to say about anyone. If somebody hurt her, she would go to her little prayer room—she had a walk-in closet in her bedroom where she'd go—she'd kneel in there sometimes for hours. If we couldn't find mama in the house and we knew she was home, we knew she was in her prayer room.

She'd come out and I'd say, "Mama, what are you doing in there?"

And she'd say, "I needed to settle some things with the Lord."

She was always so sweet and kind. Never argued with dad. Until he got into the point where he had the stroke, which was about eight years before he passed away. Then she used to lay down the law to him. He'd get pretty ornery and angry but she stayed with him right to the end. I can still see her taking care of him, washing his feet, scrubbing his back, taking him places in the automobile—all those things a good, lovely wife accepts. That "better or for worse thing." It was true with her. She was a straight-down-the-line woman. Her vows were forever. And that's what made my mother a good mother.

She lived very modestly and at times she was too modest. She was modest about herself as well. Until one day when I brought her home from the nursing home ... I knew that she wasn't happy there, so I said, "Mama, I'll take you home but you gotta help me. If you don't help me, I can't keep you home."

And she said, "I'll try my best."

I took her home on a Monday. On Wednesday, she said, "I've got to take a bath. Do you know anybody that can help me?"

I said, "I can help you." Well she didn't want me to help because I was her son. But I said, "Certainly I can. Get in your bedroom, I'll run the water, we'll get through it."

She had a big mirror on her wall so once she was dressed, she could check her appearance. Well, anyway, I told her, "Mama, the bath is ready to go."

She said, "Now don't you look at me. I'll be in but don't you look at me."

She was standing there in front of that mirror stark naked. I could see her in the glass. I said, "Mama, I see everything that you got. I can see right there in the mirror."

"Well, I guess you've seen it all." And she came walking out with her robe in her hand. So we got her into the bathtub, got her washed. That broke the ice.

I believe I'm living about six years beyond what the Bible says and I think I'm very fortunate. As far as my general health goes, I don't think it's too bad. I had a couple of broken legs. A compound fracture of one and a broken leg on the other. That was due to one motorcycle accident and an accident in the fire department. I don't really think of those as life-threatening.

I had a heart attack, a double bypass. When they took me to the hospital, I didn't even really think about it. While they were working on me, I didn't give death a thought. I could see all their faces staring down at me and the injections of all that sort of stuff and I never really thought about dying.

The colon cancer wasn't really too traumatic. I have a wonderful doctor and I'm sure things will come out all right. If it doesn't, I'm ready to go. I don't sit around and worry about it coming back. My worries are the people I love who are sick.

Life to me is focused on *learning all the time.* Everything I've done has taught me something about life. My past experiences have helped me get on with life. When something breaks or gets out of order or goes wrong or I don't know what to do, I ask myself, "What did I do the last time?" Or, "Who can come over and help me?"

I think it's important to talk to other people. We really have to communicate with feeling and touch, things such as that. You'd be surprised how far it can go when you say something nice to someone that you really mean. You can just see their face shine.

When someone does something for me, I appreciate it and I tell them. I tell them how good they are and how much I love them. Tell them how much the things they've given me or done for me mean. People shouldn't have to wait until they're dead to have nice things said about them.

*Shortly after he was interviewed, he was driving home from an appointment and had another heart attack. He quickly pulled into a gas station and told the attendant to call 911. He knew he wasn't going to make it and asked the attendant to tell his family that he loved them.*

## *Pat*

**Multiple ailments and caregiver for husband, Vic**

> *I remember thinking, "I wonder if his time is here and how much time we have." ...I remember just enough for that thought to cross my mind, "I wonder how much time we have left together."*

**[About her husband's passing]** ... It was Vic, my husband's, fortieth class reunion in Wichita, Kansas and he said he was going. I wasn't really feeling up to it ... but he wanted to go to this reunion and he wanted to drive. He told me one day he was going with or without me. I knew he was serious and if he had a pack, a shirt, and some pants that he would get in that van and start driving. I knew he might not make it all the way, but he was going to try. So of course, I chose to go along.

So we went to Wichita. He started out at the University of Wichita which was obviously the highlight in his life. We started out there. From there we went to where he played baseball where the farm team had an eye on him when he was a junior. And then the summer before his senior year, he got polio. That ended his baseball career. So we went and took pictures of all those places. Every park that he played in, every house he lived in, they were all still there but one. The place where his dad worked. Every place that you could think of. Every school that he went to, we took pictures of it all.

Then to Arkansas where he was born. He wanted to find his grandmother's grave. So we were literally in a truck going through these woods where there was just an overgrown path of weeds. We were driving through all this brush and driving through creeks in this guy's truck. [Laughs at the memory.]

He was going back to his roots.

We came back, got the pictures developed and got a bunch of albums. He was going to start working on it. We got them all numbered and named—he went through everything. I was wishing as he went through all of this that the kids could be with us. I wanted them to see where their roots came from….

We left on the second or third of October and got back on the fifth of November. But when he came back, it was really funny. It was almost surreal .... All I can remember is I can't really say whether there was anything said or not said or not done. But we came back, resumed our lives, but something was different.

I remember thinking, "I wonder if his time is here and I wonder how much time we have." He would sit on the end of his bed and it was easiest for me to go and sit on the floor and hug his legs. That's what I remember, hugging his legs. I kept thinking, "I wonder how much time we have left together."

I also prayed that I wouldn't wake up and find him in the morning, expired. I didn't want him to be driving and have an accident. I don't know why, but I didn't want the family around the bed doing the hospital scene—it just wasn't his style. I remember praying, "God I don't know what's left. What other scenario is left?"

And then ... God created one. It was so final. He wanted to die in the blink of an eye—and he did. There was no recovering him. Everybody ... the finest medical help was there immediately. But he was gone.

*Vic died at his rehabilitation gym—suddenly and peacefully.*

**[About her chronic and acute health battles] ...**

The primary illness that keeps me from living a normal life would be the fibromyalgia—that's the fatigue, pain, and brain fog. I find that a lot of people don't know what that is. It becomes immobilizing in the sense that you have to lay down. Your brain just stops on you. The pain is all-encompassing. You try to focus away from it, but it's immobilizing—literally and figuratively. You lose everything of yourself, identity and everything.

Every once in a while, I haul out the collage my daughter made of my life for me and say, "Yea, this is me. I'm still this person. It doesn't feel like it right now, but I'm still this person."

Now, I'm feeling like my life is totally out of control because of my health. Knowing I have to make changes, not sure how to read those changes. And not wanting to make those changes, wanting to keep things the same.

When I was laying in the emergency room the first time—so dizzy and weak and could hardly talk—I thought I might be having a stroke. It felt like, like some people say they feel, like you're going to die. I was so incapacitated. You are just totally out of control of everything. I was laying there and realizing that I was completely in God's hands. You realize from having lost a spouse that there is that blink of an eye from this world to the next. You feel like you're at the doorstep and you don't know what's going to happen. I did have a sense that it was my time but I wasn't sure—and I didn't care.

Then, the second time, when I went in paralyzed, it was like, "OK, I'm paralyzed, this is possibly a stroke but people do recuperate. I got here early."

My body was partially paralyzed. I could move from the left to the right side, but not from the right to the left. I was thrown into this place where I was dependent for everything, from somebody else. It's something I'll never forget. And then in the subsequent days, every day, I realized all that I used to do for myself, now takes a myriad of people to do it for me. It's unbelievable.

The following testimonies were added when the Second Edition was published. They have a different tone because they weren't transcribed from interviews; they were published essays, chapters in memoirs, or dictated testimonies. Each person was invited to participate in the Second Edition and gave written consent for their story to be included.

### *Sharon Coble*

**A testimony she shared regarding the power of reading God's Word out loud to her grandmother when she was hospitalized as a hospice patient ...**

In 1976, my paternal grandmother was in the hospital, dying from advanced age and infirmities. She had been a pastor's wife for over fifty years but none of the people caring for her knew of her background—they didn't know that she had read the Word of God every day of her life from the time she could read….

By the time my brother, Devan, and I arrived to see her, she had been in the hospital a week or so. She had not been able to read or hear God's Word for the first time in all those years. She looked like a dry desert, dying for lack of water. We began reading the Bible to her, starting in Genesis, each of us at a pace of two hours for an average of eight hours a day. Although she was in a coma, she would often lick her lips as if she were drinking cool, clear water. She knew the Word by heart, so we didn't leave out a single verse.

By the time she passed away a week or so later, she had come out of her coma and recognized the people around her. The power of God's Word to nourish and strengthen us is mighty! Only God knows how many people will come to know Him through the simple reading of His Words.

*Curt was touched that people were praying for him to be healed.... but, he said very emphatically, "Don't pray that I'll be healed, pray that God will use my life however many days are left."*

## *Curt Kraft*

**With his wife Mary by his side**

I'm more of a listener than a talker now. Oxygen is helping a lot. This recliner lets me get into just the right position where I don't have pressure on my liver ... it lets me lay back. People are welcome to come over. I like to see people, talk to them—but, I get so tired. I just don't have the energy to talk anymore. I enjoy it when company comes and I can just sit here and listen. The cancer, the pressure is here in my lungs. I don't have the volume to get my words out anymore.

To go back to the beginning ... I was working on the house like a mule. I was digging this bank out here. I was hauling dirt in the wheelbarrow. Taking it across the street to the neighbor's yard. In fact, at first, I told Mary that I thought I'd pulled a muscle right here [points to area below his right breastbone]. I had a little bit of pain and thought it was from pushing the wheelbarrow. But the doctor later diagnosed it as Stage Four cancer in the liver, lungs, skeleton, and neck.

I'd have to say I was completely shocked that I was really sick! I'd thought maybe it was my gall bladder or something simple ... I wasn't weak, I just had this pain. In fact, part of the tests came back 'outstanding'. That's the strange part, I had Stage Four cancer when I found out ... but I'd just had my blood work done and it showed my liver was working perfectly. The cancer was already in my liver, lungs, skeleton, and brain. It was everywhere.

They told me, "We give you six months without chemo and maybe two years with chemo." Basically, they were saying there was no cure but they might be able to prolong my life. That's why they call this a 'silent killer' because when you finally find out about it, it's too late. There's no test you could take and see what's going on.

A little bit before that, Mary and I wanted to have a Bible Study in our home. We felt God blessed us with this house and we wanted to make use of it—whether it was downstairs, on the deck, or upstairs here. So ... we had this Bible Study with six couples and called ourselves the Twelve Disciples. We wanted to start off with something easy to understand ... I'd really enjoyed *The Purpose Driven Life,* so we decided to use that. We would read a chapter each week and just talk about it. Something as simple as that! We made it through the first six chapters and then everyone was going on vacation, so we decided to take a break and start back up in the fall.

Two weeks after we took the break, I got this diagnosis. But, God was so gentle with me. I kept thinking of the first six chapters of *The Purpose Driven Life* and the very first sentence is—"It's not about me." It helped me not put the emphasis on me or the cancer, it's all about GOD. It hit me so strongly that we're just pilgrims passing through … life is a gift. He kept working on me to think about what was really important and not concentrate on the cancer.

People say to me, "I don't understand how you can go through all of this and still trust God." It's because I've surrendered. It's all about knowing God has a plan and a purpose for my life. We can't lean on our own understanding. We're never going to be able to understand what God is doing. We have to surrender to God and know He's in control of everything.

I never really felt like, "Woe is me" or "Why did this happen to me?" I always have felt like my cup is half full instead of half empty. I've always felt that Mary and I have been overly blessed. Why did God choose us to be blessed in so many different ways? I mean, 60 years—that's a long time! That is a good life!

I'd say my faith comes from ... I had the benefit of growing up with just an amazing mother … she's just a rock-solid Christian. She 'walks the talk' more than any other Christian I know. No matter which family member you talk to from Oregon to Minnesota to Florida to California, they would all immediately say the same thing—she's just an amazing person. I had the benefit of having her as a mother to guide and lead me … whatever actions I was doing when I was young … I was always guided by, "Would this make my mom proud?"

There was one time … I was in the shower and I was thinking … I was having a conversation with God and saying, "God, I just wanted to be the best grandpa in the whole world. That was my goal."

And immediately, it was one of those times when I could hear His voice. He said, "You ARE being the best grandpa in the whole world because you're teaching your grandkids to trust and obey me."

I got chills. I thought, "Well, that's the end of the conversation." [Laughs.]

He was right, I was teaching them to trust and obey Him. I always planned to take them to the Big Trees Park and … teach them how to identify plants and flowers. I wanted to do all of these things that I'd done with the Junior Rangers in the past, during my 30-year park career. After the diagnosis, I was thinking I was going to miss out on that. I felt like God was saying, "Don't worry about it, that's a worldly thing. That's of THIS world. It's much more important to teach them to trust and obey me!"

There are times like that … where God has spoken to me and I know He's right beside me. I had an experience one day when I was in a park … I sensed His presence right next to me at the table. He was right there with me, giving me strength and courage. When you have experiences like that, it's hard to explain or transfer that to someone else—they almost have to have the experience themselves—you can't just tell them,

"Well, you should believe in God because He sat next to me at a picnic table." But, if you had that experience yourself, then you know that you know that you know. That's where I'm at. You want to be the best witness you could possibly be for God. Glorify His name. Give Him all the honor and praise for anything that comes at you.

I can see Him working … I see Him bringing souls toward Him. Even in this circumstance—I'm amazed and in awe of His grace … to step back and see Him working through all of this stuff.

Of course, it's a lot easier for me than it is for Mary and the rest of the family. But … we're working together as a team, just like we always have. I told Mary, "We're a team." She's such a great example of a devoted wife—serving her husband. It's difficult for her but she's a great caregiver, devoted to her husband. I always knew that about her. So, it didn't surprise me when it came down to this most trying of circumstances, she would be there like she always has been.

This whole last year that we've had … that's where I've been finding joy, even with all the trials and tribulations. Before this, I never understood James 1:2—How can you have joy when you're going through trials and tribulations? Why would you be happy? Now I can see it because there have been so many joyful moments in the last year. The joy has come BECAUSE of the trials and tribulations.

I got to meet so many of my goals in the last year: got to visit my 50$^{th}$ state, had my 40$^{th}$ wedding anniversary, got to play basketball at my 60$^{th}$ birthday party, got to take a road trip with the grandchildren to The Heritage Farm in South Dakota ... so many ways to be blessed.

So many people have come closer to God because of my trial. I've gotten many letters and cards and notes with deep heartfelt thoughts. Mary and I realize that God has been so gentle with me in the face of this diagnosis.

I said this once in a talk I gave at a family reunion, and it has become so very real throughout the last year: We have hope in Him who offers promises of a heavenly reward.

*Curt passed away peacefully, in his home, surrounded by the family and friends he loved on January 14, 2008, 15 months after his diagnosis.*

***Beverly Schroeder-McConnell***

[Excerpts from her life review manuscript]

**Caregiver to two husbands, Paul and Owen**

**Paul's death.**

Paul passed away suddenly on his birthday—I always thought he would die doing something dangerous and he did. He was a daredevil, that's what his family thought too. He was riding a snowmobile and died tragically on his birthday.

Sometimes I rode with Paul and the boys but I didn't go on that trip. I was at the cabin [California Sierra's] making a birthday dinner with a birthday cake. I heard the sirens going on and on and it kind of went through me that someone must have gotten hurt up country. Hours later, two men in yellow slickers came in and told me that Paul died. Craig was with him when he died. I just collapsed, fell right to the floor … I can see that moment like it was yesterday.

I kept saying, "But it's his birthday!"

I turned the prime rib off and … well, I don't think we even had dinner that night. It was such a traumatic event.

My pastor from Calvary (Pine Grove, CA) came over to the cabin to talk with us. Pastor George led Paul's service and he did such a good, personal job. The boys both wrote a little thing and got up to speak. I couldn't do it but they did. I was like a Zombie.

After that, my sons said, "Come on mom, we're going back to Redwood City."

I got in the car like they told me to and didn't even think about what I was doing or where we were going.

I was in shock for a long time. Then, I was criticized for going back to work too early because I just didn't want to sit home and rethink everything. I didn't want to be home alone. I'd never been alone! From my parent's home, I went into marriage … it was hard to suddenly be by myself.

I worked through it but didn't get therapy for Craig and I probably should have (Kirk was older and wasn't there the weekend Paul died). The first or second night after Paul died, I could hear Craig in the back bedroom sobbing and I just held him. I think that changed him and I wish I would have gotten some help for him. Back then, you just didn't think about getting counseling for things like this. You just thought that somehow you'd get over it.

I got depressed too. One day I decided I wasn't going to get up, I was going to stay in bed all day. In fact, I spent one day in bed and felt so crummy the next day, I thought *I'm never doing this again, it's not in my vocabulary*. So I'd go shopping instead, I didn't need to buy anything, I just needed to get out of the house. I figured, if you want to throw a pity party, no one is going to want to join you! I knew Paul wouldn't want me to sit home and feel sorry for myself.

I went to a therapist for a while ... I guess it helped. He kept asking me what I felt and I'd tell him (the therapist) about everyone else. And he'd say, "But what are YOU feeling?" I couldn't tell him about my feelings because I didn't think I had any. He kept working with me so I could get in touch with how I felt.

I went back to work ... had things I had to do, business to take care of. I had contracts and needed to fulfill them. For me, that was a good choice.

I put on a good facade because I had to be a professional in my job, but that didn't mean I was doing good! I didn't run around with red eyes and a Kleenex in my hand! I did my crying in private.

I'll never forget this ... after Paul died and I had to change all the names on everything, ... my friend at the title company told me that I had to sign as an unmarried woman. I remember crying and saying, "I don't want to be unmarried!"

**Owen**

I was only 57 years old when Paul died, too young to just give up on companionship. But, it was two years before I even started thinking about dating.

My friend introduced me to Owen ... we knew we were being set up for a blind date. We went to dinner with some of my childhood friends [in Michigan] and were introduced. I was a nervous wreck because I hadn't dated for a long time.

In walks this cute little Irishman with a grin and sparkling eyes!

It worked out really well! We stood outside the restaurant talking after dinner because we had so much in common! We grew up in the same community and knew many of the same people [Petoskey, Michigan].

So Owen and I were dating, flying back and forth across the country for our dates. We had to get tickets to fly back and forth—back then, airfare was really cheap. We decided that we were either going to have to buy the airline or get married.

I married Owen on May 15th, 1995. Owen Dwight McConnell. His birthday was March 30, 1930. He died August 1, 2007.

The year Owen died ... he was getting pretty frail. I noticed that he was moving really, really slow. He thought he needed more exercise and joined a gym. Neither of us had a clue about how serious it was.

One Saturday, we went to a function downtown, some sort of festival in the spring. He said his back hurt and he would sit down as often as he could and then get up and keep going. I didn't think too much about it.

On Sunday, he slept almost all day. I noticed because it was so unlike him—he was always up and about, always doing something.

Monday morning, I called the doctor early and told him I thought something was wrong. We went in and the doctor came out to talk to me almost in tears, he thought a lot of Owen.

He said, "I'm so sorry, I hate to tell you this, but Owen has Acute Myelogenous Leukemia. He's got ten days or maybe two months to live."

I didn't tell Owen right away—I didn't know how to tell someone he was going to die in a little while. How do you do that? I was in shock.

Finally, I told him, "I have to tell you this, I'm not really happy about it, but I have to tell you…."

He looked at me and said, "You know, I've lived a really good life, I've had three good wives and the last one was the best! I don't have any regrets."

So he was calm and okay with it. I guess maybe he knew but he hadn't said anything to me.

That Friday night, he got a fever. The doctor said to take him to the ER and they admitted him to the hospital. I was afraid he was going to bleed out at home so I was glad he was there and they could take care of him.

He went into the hospital on a Friday night and died the following Wednesday. He was to the point where he couldn't get out of bed. It was that quick—the doctor was right, ten days.

I was over there all the time. Exhausted. His daughter said she would come and stay the night with him so I could go home and get some sleep.

I went home to rest and … apparently about six in the morning, he asked her where I was because he wanted to talk to me. She told him I was at home resting. I wish she would have called me. By the time I got there, probably about 6:30, he was in a coma and I never got a chance to talk to him before he died.

My sister was there to help me deal with the loss. My kids were with me. You just do it. I have some blank spots in my memory because it happened so fast and I was in shock. The doctor told me that most people don't survive that kind of cancer and he knew Owen wouldn't either. He was supposed to have radiation but he died before it started. They knew it wouldn't save him but when you're presented with something that sounds like hope, you take it.

He died very, very peacefully, just went to sleep. I heard him make a little noise and then I called the nurse. I told her, "I think he's gone." And she said, "Yes, he is."

He died about 3 in the afternoon. No pain, he just went to sleep.

## *Carolyne Winter*

**Carolyne buried two of her adult children**

*For the full stories of Gay Lynne and Danny,*
*See "A Winter's Remembrance",*
*by Carolyne Winter, available on Amazon.*
***This short testimony was written for a guest column on a website.***

Gay Lynn was 23 years old. Our daughter's dream to be a game warden was just months away. The love of her life had proposed and wedding plans were imminent.

However, instead of moving into an exciting phase of life, she stood in the rain at the side of Highway 1 trying to flag down a patrol car. Something was wrong. She didn't know what but knew she needed help. Quickly.

California Highway Patrol Officer Castle did stop to help. He wrapped her in his jacket and rushed her to an emergency room just two miles away in San Luis Obispo.

We never saw her wear a warden's uniform or walk down the aisle in white … But, we did sit by her bedside for twelve brutal days while she fought for her life.

Gay Lynn had experienced a massive intracranial bleed from an aneurysm. There was no cure. There would be no path to healing from all the destruction left in its wake.

After a long night of relentless seizures left her comatose, she looked as if she had been through a war zone. Her hospital gown and sheets were crumpled, her long blonde hair matted and damp with perspiration.

My mind and heart were shattered. She was on a ventilator but 'she' was already gone.

A nurse we hadn't seen before walked into my hopeless moment.

Nurse Penny put her hands on her hips and declared, "Oh, Miss Gay Lynn, you look like hell. It's time for a bath."

This kind-beyond-measure nurse proceeded to bathe our daughter from head to toe. She refreshed the bed with new sheets and dressed our daughter in her prettiest nightgown. Then, she carefully brushed her hair and gathered it into a pretty top knot.

It was the most beautiful thing a stranger could have done for Gay Lynn and us. We knew the end was near, but Nurse Penny took the time to show caring and respect for our beautiful daughter's body.

Jesus came for Gay Lynn four days later.

.....

People ask: How did you do it? How did you bury your firstborn child, your only daughter, without giving in to despair?

I confess, there were days I didn't do it very well.

In the beginning … I tried to lean on my faith, but it was easier to find relief in the bottom of a wine bottle.

Eventually, God's grace won. My sons needed ***me*** in the land of the living (not just a functioning body). I set the bottle aside and turned to Jesus for help. Step-by-step, He showed me the way and never left my side … He insulated me from the full force of grief while pulling me closer to Him.

I learned many things through her death and the aftermath:

> When our Godly assignments are completed on earth, He takes us to be with Him. Whatever Gay Lynn was born to do, she did. He numbered her days before she was even born and came for her when those days were complete. *Ecclesiastes 3:1-2, Job 14:5, Psalm 139*
>
> My faith was tested and then strengthened by this truth: My thoughts are not His thoughts and my plans are not His plans. *Isaiah 55:8-9*

I still miss Gay Lynn and will as long as I live. One day, I'll see her again. She'll be gloriously restored and alive. I yearn for that day. And, when it comes, I know I'll see her then like I never could this side of heaven. *Revelation 21:1-4*

## *Sylvia Johnson*

**Caregiver for her husband, Gerry**

This story is from her memoir,

*The Book Of Sylvia*
Sylvia Johnson, 2023.
Excerpts from the chapter entitled: The Gift, pages 111-123

In March of 2003, I arrived home from work one afternoon and Gerry said he'd gone to our family doctor and had him look at something under his tongue.

The doctor was concerned and referred Gerry to a head and neck specialist in Lodi [California]. This doctor took one look under Gerry's tongue and said, "You have cancer."

If you think that was any indication of his so-called bedside manner, you're right! Very abrupt, very gruff and just not a nice person. Gerry didn't care. He just wanted it treated and eliminated.

We prayed that God would give us peace knowing He was in control of all that would evolve.

The first year was comprised of surgery to remove part of his tongue, chemotherapy and radiation. For a few weeks during radiation (two trips a day, an hour one way), to Lodi were necessary. He and I would drive down to Lodi for a 7:30 AM appointment and return home. In the afternoon I would drive him to Jackson where he would board a cancer van which took him to an afternoon treatment. This was five days a week for several weeks.

I couldn't work and be a caregiver at the same time, so I retired from the mortgage and loan business.

. . . . .

Due to his illness Gerry and I were together all the time, which truly was a blessing.

We treated the trips to the doctors or for treatments as outings. We both felt so powerless over everything going on, our behavior changed in a lot of areas.

One area was I started automatically praying out loud in the car as we were on our way to an appointment and on the way home. If the news was encouraging, I praised the Lord. If the news was discouraging, I'd pray for the Lord to help us get through this.

Gerry would always end my prayer with a verbal, "Amen"!!

The head and neck specialist from Lodi would come to Jackson to treat patients one day a week. In March of 2004, after a year of treatment, Gerry had an appointment with him to hear the results of his latest tests. His strength and energy were at levels that allowed him to drive to Jackson (15 minutes) to meet with the doctor on a Thursday morning.

I came home from Bible Study just before noon to find Gerry had returned from his appointment. He was literally circling our dining table.

I said, “What’s wrong?!?!”

He hesitantly said, “The doctor told me to go home and get my things in order.”

“What? What does that mean?” I said in total disbelief.

After a few minutes, I asked Gerry if I should call our pastor. We called, and he was over to our house within 15 minutes.

After he and Gerry talked for just a minute or so, our pastor said, “We’re all going to die, Gerry, you just have a better idea of when.”

Was I feeling full of faith at that moment? Not really. I was feeling fear. *What will Gerry have to endure? Will I be able to care for him? What about finances?* And the list goes on.

Pastor prayed with us and came to visit several times. On one of his visits, he brought his traveling communion set as well as his wife (who I knew well) and the four of us had communion together. By observing communion and praying together, our faith was strengthened, and any fears we might have melted away.

We drew close to God as we placed our lives in His hands. I would read the Bible to Gerry in the evening. We also read devotional books and books on heaven from trusted authors. My daughter found a great DVD on heaven. What an experience to be able to learn about heaven with someone who knew they would be going there within a short period of time.

Oddly enough, even though one might have cancer, you still must take care of the rest of your body. Consequently, Gerry was due for a visit to his Cardiologist, Doctor C. in Lodi. We both loved this man! He shared with us that when he first became a doctor, he thought he was God! He explained that people treated him this way… even at social gatherings. Then his sister became very ill, and he *just knew* she would not die. He was a doctor! She died.

Doctor C. was completely devastated. Because he was raised in a Christian home, and due to his family's influence, he began attending church with them. Eventually, he turned his life over to the Lord.

He was a great encouragement to Gerry. After our last visit there, he walked out in the waiting room with Gerry and as Gerry opened the door to leave, he said, “I’ll see you in heaven, Gerry.”

Gerry answered, "I'll be waiting."

.....

By March of 2005, Gerry had been in hospice for six months. The nurse, Mary, came by for her weekly visit. She and Gerry had become friends. She was interested in airplanes, a subject Gerry could talk about for hours, having spent four years in the Air Force.

One day when she came, I followed her into the bedroom. Gerry was propped up on pillows and smiled at her as she sat down on the chair beside him.

I was standing at the foot of the bed.

After greeting each other she said, "Gerry, I'm going to ask you some questions about common occurrences during this stage of your illness. Have you seen visions of family members or past friends who have passed away?"

He shook his head that he had not. (Talking at this point had become very difficult.) She continued, "Have you seen any angels?" As he slowly processed this, he lifted his right arm and pointed at me.

Wow! Tears came to my eyes, and I said, "Gerry, I will never forget this moment." And I haven't. It was the greatest gift he could have ever left with me.

I say this because being a caregiver is a very difficult position. You get frustrated, you feel helpless at times, and you find yourself just plain worn out. Certainly, I said things in a tone of voice that was less than loving, took out some of my frustration on him and had behavior that was less than angelic. But he chose not to remember those times and saw me in a positive and loving way.

By doing so he erased the possibility of any future guilt on my part.

Mary was leaving and I followed her out to her car.

She said Gerry had about a week and outlined what I could expect. It was overwhelming. I told her I wasn't a nurse, and up to this point I hadn't been exposed to anything even close to what she was saying. She assured me a nurse was always available.

After she left, I checked on Gerry, and he was ready for a nap. I let him know I was going on my walk, and I would be back within half an hour.

There's a beautiful trail amongst the trees at the bottom of our driveway. I was on the trail calling out loud to the Lord, "You know I'm not equipped to deal with what's going to happen!"

I felt I needed to let Him know. Of course He knew! Of course He would equip me!

. . . . .

That was March 10, and on March 12, a Saturday, I received a call from Doctor H., our primary doctor, who needed to check on Gerry before signing the paperwork extending Hospice care. He asked if he could come over that evening. Gerry looked forward to his visit.

Doctor H. sat in a chair by the bed, asked Gerry how he was doing, and chatted for a while. Gerry listened and nodded his head.

After a few minutes he said, "You know, Gerry, it's okay to let go."

Gerry immediately turned his head and looked at me.

I quietly said, "It's true, Gerry, it's okay."

The next day Gerry died in his sleep. It was March 13, 2005. It had been only three days since the nurse's visit, not a week, and Gerry did not have to experience any of the painful and undignified symptoms the nurse had mentioned might occur.

. . . . .

It's been 18 years since his departure. I'm surprised how often I think of him and the gift he left me just a couple of days before he died, by pointing his finger at me when the hospice nurse asked if he'd *'seen any angels'*. I am forever grateful, Gerry.

### *Betty Fisher*

**Caregiver for her husband, Butch**

*[Betty's oral testimony was typed into a document.]*

Technically, Butch was never a hospice patient nor was I ever his full-time caregiver. But, I was by his side when he went through two years of chemotherapy to beat non-Hodgkins lymphoma. And, I was standing next to his bed when he took his last breath.

He'd successfully endured all the treatments and had just been declared cancer-free. In typical Butch style, he walked up and down the street with his arms in the air saying, "I beat it, I beat it." He made the whole neighborhood smile as we celebrated his victory with him.

Little did we guess that just two months later, he'd get COVID and die within days. In so many, many ways, a heartbreaking end to a life well-lived.

We'd been to a party with friends on a Saturday night. Sunday morning, Butch woke up sick and decided to take a COVID test. We both tested positive. By the end of that day, I'd driven him to the ER for the first time. They sent him home with instructions to treat it like the flu.

I took him to the ER again the next day ... by then it was pneumonia. They sent him home.

The third day, he had back spasms, excruciating pain, and was disoriented. Looking back, I believe his organs were already shutting down. I called 911 and they took him to the ER for me.

By that night, doctors admitted it was too late for a good outcome. We were allowed to be with him in a special room at the hospital (me, both of our kids, and our grandson). And then ... the man with a huge heart ... the idea man who was always ready to entertain or travel with friends ... husband, father, grandfather, brother, uncle, friend to hundreds—was gone. Gone from every place but our memories.

In the beginning, I was sick with COVID and frozen by the unexpected grief and loss. People told me I handled his death gracefully but I was just trying to get through the days and nights the best I knew how. My faith, family, and long-time friends gave me comfort throughout those rough days.

I also had a new group of friends from the neighborhood we'd just moved to. I will be forever grateful to the Callaway Lane Ladies who reached out to me in my time of need. They found so many ways to be there for me: cards, words of comfort, food when I had out-of-state family for Butch's celebration of life, as well as our weekly get-together for Bible Study and prayer. I thank the good Lord daily for putting me on this block with these friends. I have been blessed.

A month after Butch died, we were able to honor his life with an outdoor celebration attended by many family and friends. We were fortunate and blessed ... in those early days of COVID, many people died alone in the hospital because no one was allowed to touch you or say goodbye. And, celebration of life gatherings were taboo. God helped us in both of those regards.

After the legal paperwork was filed, the service finished, thank-you notes sent ... I felt fresh waves of loss all over again. This time it seemed to cut a little deeper. I knew I had to find something to occupy my mind and hands, so I looked for things to do.

The reason I've agreed to participate in this hospice book is that I did find several projects to help me process my heartache. They were tangible things I could do and paved the way for comfort and even some smiles. Yes, they also inspired a river or two of tears ... but even those times opened the door for the healing process to begin.

Whenever we traveled, Butch would buy a t-shirt as a souvenir. I had drawers and shelves full of his shirts. I decided to transform some of his special t-shirts into pillows for family. Working with the stretchy fabric was challenging but I figured out a pattern, persevered, and got each one done. Of the ten I made, some had to be mailed and some were passed out in person.

I still had many nice shirts left and decided to sew them into a lap quilt. Something I could cuddle up with while I watched TV or read. I did need help with that and found a company to make it for me.

Then, I started sorting all the cards I'd received after Butch passed. So many beautiful cards and words ... I wanted to preserve them and make it easy to reread them whenever I needed to. I started creating a scrapbook album with color-coordinated pages and extra information. It took a long time to finish but I'm so glad I did. On my blue days, I get it out and go through it, reading the things people told me and the stories they shared. Rather than make me sadder, it gives me comfort.

[An added smile, after Butch died, I found a Valentine's card I'd given him in 1988. For some reason, he'd put it in the glove box of his truck and carried it with him wherever he went. Finding it touched me so I put it in my album of remembrances too.]

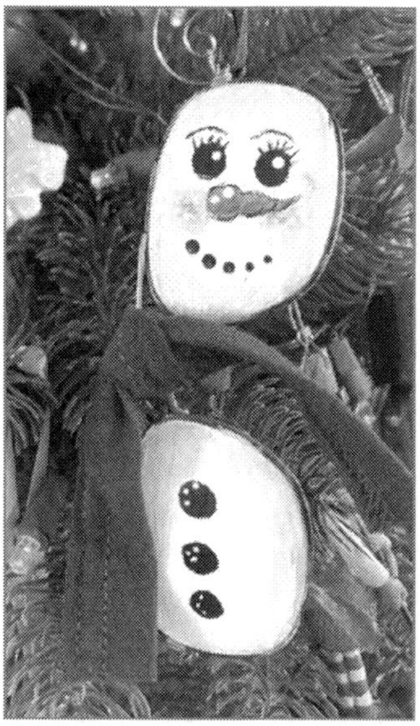

One other thing that ended up holding special meaning was finding all of his eyeglasses ... he had glasses everywhere. All kinds of colors, shapes, and sizes. I'd seen how to turn used glasses into snowman ornaments and decided to make some. With the help of a good friend (who put the finishing touches on them), I was able to turn many of them into cute tree ornaments.

The ornaments gave me another idea ... Butch was a golfer and had accumulated many golf mementos over the years (gifts or travel souvenirs). I decided to dedicate a special Christmas tree to his memory every year by using all of his golf items as decorations. I put a pair of his snowman glasses on it and use a golf glove for the 'topper'.

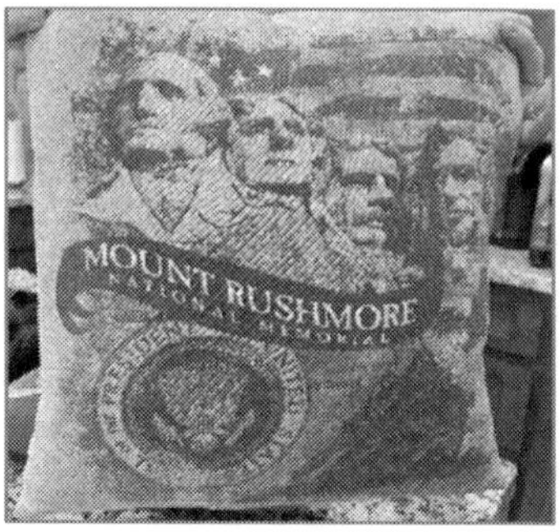


We were married 55 years when he died. He was the love of my life and I, his. I'll miss him as long as I live. I'm so grateful we did all the things we did when he was here. Those memories continue to sustain me. And, I know, someday I'll see him again in heaven. Til then, I'll treasure my memories and love him from afar.

## Therapeutic Reminiscing

**GOAL: give people an excuse to talk. Draw out their narratives in as natural a setting as possible. Record with tape recorder/pen and paper notes.**

This is the method I use when I'm conducting a life review—it's what I used to gather the above interviews as well as 40 interviews since. It's a simple, easy-to-use interview protocol that inspires reminiscing and sharing. If you would like to interview someone you care about, read the ideas listed and use what you feel would be appropriate for them.

It's best to do several short interviews with different approaches (talking, going through photos, etc.). If you give them a break between interviews, they'll start thinking of things they want to tell or show you. They may wish to retell a story they told earlier or one you've heard many times before—let them. If they repeat a story, that's a good indication that something about that story is significant to them. And, chances are, if you let them retell it at their own pace, they'll take it to a different emotional level. Also, take note of the first story they choose to tell you, something about that story holds special meaning.

Tape record everything but let them know they're being taped. At first, that may add a little awkwardness to the storytelling, but they'll soon forget about the recorder. I always keep a notepad and pen when someone tells me stories; occasionally, I write down words or phrases I find interesting or are repeated. Taking notes says, "I'm listening and what you're telling me is important."

Photograph reviews work well too. "What is this photo of? Who is in it? Where is this? Why is it one of your favorites? What is happening here? How does it make you feel to look at it now?"

On the following pages, you'll find a copy of the interview protocol I use for *Legacies.* I've included all of the questions but suggest you only use the ones that work well with your storyteller. Some added suggestions:

- Take your time, don't change subjects until you're convinced the speaker's ready to talk about something else.

- Use "silent probes": if you feel that the person hasn't told you everything/is leaving something out—don't say anything. Often after a "silent probe," individuals will share something they've wanted to say for a long time.

- Don't try to get them to tell their story in chronological order. Let them tell their stories in their own order and in their own way.

- Try to get them to recreate the moment: what did they see, smell, hear, touch, taste? How did the event make them feel?

If the person is too weak to talk, have a group of family members and friends reminisce in their presence. It will bless them to hear you talking about your memories of events in their lives. They may be able to interject comments or thoughts into stories. I tape-record these group reminiscing sessions as well. It can be a very healing time for family members … almost a precursor to the grieving process.

Don’t be afraid of tears. It doesn’t mean they’re upset; it means the memory still has the power to touch them.

## Life Review Interview:

### Part One: Life review

"I wonder if you could tell me a little bit about your life, perhaps beginning with where and when you were born…." [NOTE: Most people will tell you where and when they were born, maybe a couple of other childhood facts, and then take a huge time leap to when they got married and started their own family. I find this phenomenon interesting because, when encouraged to do so, most individuals love to talk about their childhood. If your speaker skips their childhood, gently try to coax childhood reminiscing…]

Childhood: Parent's names, occupations of parents, personalities of parents
Siblings, birth order
How would you describe your home life
Describe a typical day in your childhood
Any favorite stories about your birth or childhood
Best memories of childhood

When you grew up, what did you do:
Education… work… places you've lived
Are you married… how did you meet… years married
Do you have children, ages, gender, where do they live

[[Retired:
Grandchildren? Great-grandchildren?
Do you have any special interests or hobbies?
How do you like to spend your free time?

What do you consider your "passion?"

How would you describe your religious beliefs or spirituality to a stranger?

Most lives can be divided into different periods—circumstances or choices make your life significantly different. What were the major turning points in your life? What are the places where a biographer would probably start a new chapter?

What events in your life gave you a sense of fulfillment or pride?

Are there any events you regret?

How would you describe yourself? [They usually ask, "What do you mean?" Let them decide how to answer this question … it usually causes a little bump in the interview while they decide how to answer. This may be a good time to practice the 'silent probe' interview technique.]

If someone asked you for advice about 'living a good life' what would you tell them?
Who have been the most influential people in your life? Why?

**Part Two: Memorials**

Let's go back to some of the occasions and people that you talked about earlier and consider more questions (events, passions, hobbies, work, religious beliefs, influential people, moments of pride, regret, etc.).

Do you have any items to remind yourself of ___

Where do you keep it?

Who knows why you keep it?

What do you hope will happen to it when you're no longer here?

I'm going to mention some ways that other people have marked or memorialized their lives and then ask if you have participated in any of these activities as well...

Do you take pictures? What do you do with them?

Do you keep scrapbooks about yourself or people you care about?

Do keep diaries or journals?

Have you, or has anyone who knows you, ever made a video of your life?

Do you have a portfolio of your work or educational accomplishments?

Do you have any copyrighted work?

Do you collect things?

What do you consider your greatest treasure?

Why is it valuable?

Where do you keep it or them (assuming it's not people)?

Who knows how valuable it is to you?

What is your favorite place in your home?

Why? What makes this your favorite place?

What does this room say about you?

If we were to bury a time capsule today with the idea that in 100 years your descendants will be looking at what's inside, what would you put inside of it to show them what your life was like, who you were, or the people you loved? Picture a container the size of a shoebox.

# Appendix

Scriptures in alphabetical order

For more information about ***Legacies***

http://www.BonnieEvansLegacies.com

bonniere@gmail.com

***Legacies***

*Preserving Memories of Ordinary People*

Ione. California

## *Other Works by This Author:*

Available on Amazon

***Blooming In The Dark, Second Edition***
*Hope For Those Going Through Hard Times*

The stories, photography, poetry, inspirational thoughts, and prayers in this book are filled with encouragement for those trying to grow in hard soil or dim light. The words of hope were gleaned from the author's seasons of darkness and—more importantly—from the unrelenting sweetness of God's presence through it all.

***Come, Let's Reason Together***
*A Biblical and Reflective Look at God's Questions*

This reflective Bible study examines eight biblical questions and the core Christian principles each represents. Each chapter is self-contained and can be completed in any order a participant or group decides is best.

***One Thing I Know…***
*How To Write An Effective & Balanced Testimony*

Through a step-by-step process, this workbook helps participants document God's interventions in their lives. (The book can be used by any participant or in a workshop setting. Contact the author for more information.)

***The Forever Love Of God***
*Before Genesis, Beyond Revelation*

The Bible has hundreds of themes woven throughout its pages. The author of this small book follows the scarlet thread of His unconditional love. You're invited to watch His love unfold through stories of creation, the fall of humanity, God's plan for redemption, and the promise of paradise.

***He Loves You More** …*
*Letters to my daughter*

This inspirational book offers encouragement to those facing public harassment or bullying on social media platforms. It includes text messages, Bible verses, prayers, short sayings, as well as journaling pages with prompts for the reader.

*Bonnie Evans is a published author as well as a Bible study teacher, speaker, and workshop facilitator. Since God revealed Himself to her in 1974, He's walked with her through many blessed and challenging seasons. He's called, commissioned, and anointed her to be an encourager for others, especially those going through long seasons of hard times.*

bonniere@gmail.com
http://www.BonnieEvansLegacies.com

Made in the USA
Las Vegas, NV
30 December 2025

38240541R00079